Healing Medicine

To Ron

Stan Blake

January 2006

Also by Steve Blake:

Alternative Remedies

Medicinal Plant Names

Herbal Property Dictionary

Nutrient Wizard CD-ROM

Natural Healing Solutions

Aromatherapy and Essential Oils

Chinese Patent Remedies

Ayurvedic Remedies

Medicinal Plant Actions

Constituents of Medicinal Plants

Medicinal Plant Constituents

Herbal Medicine CD-ROM

Natural Remedies for All

PlanetHerb CD-ROM

GlobalHerb

Healing Medicine

A Consumer's Guide to Safer Medicine

STEVE BLAKE

LifeLong Press
Haiku, Maui

LifeLong Press
http://www.NaturalHealthWizards.com
355 Honopou Road
Haiku, Maui, HI 96708

Printed in the United States of America

Cover Art by Catherine Blake

Dedication

This book is dedicated to two of my best teachers, Bernard Jensen and Robert K. M. Cooper.

It is also dedicated to my wife, Catherine. Her knowledge and intelligence have been invaluable in the preparation of this book.

Acknowledgments

I wish to thank the following people for their review and comments: Martha Sasser, Chris Meletis, Carolyn Willard, John Robbins, Charles Inlander, Michael Tierra, Michael on Red Shift, Karim Wingedheart, Debbie Carvalko, Judy Nelson, Eduardo Rincon-Gallardo, Samuel Epstein, Ivan Illich, Ruth Winter, Paul Stitt, and Dean Black.

Contents

Introduction

Over one trillion dollars is spent on health in America every year. In spite of this, Americans are in poor health. The current epidemics are heart and circulatory disease, cancer, arthritis, diabetes, and other chronic diseases. Modern medicine needs more emphasis on true prevention and on finding safe, long-term cures for these diseases. There is significant damage done to people and society by the chemicals and devices of medicine.

Medicine in America has taken a wrong turn. We need to create a new medicine. The solution is to include more treatment options than just drugs and surgery. We need to learn how to support healing which is a different approach than manipulating our bodies with powerful chemicals. We also need to learn how to prevent disease rather than trying to cure disease after it develops.

Diseases are, in many cases, created by the lifestyles of the people who get them and the environments in which they live. It takes many years for a chronic disease to develop. We can choose our food and activity levels. We can sometimes avoid stress and environmental chemicals. We can take control of our own health. We have the opportunity to find out how to live so that we can achieve excellent health. I have seen that people who practice optimum health habits are seldom bothered by disease. This book will guide you toward optimum health and disease resistance.

For too long medicine has been missing the deeper causes of disease and drugging us to suppress our symptoms. Informed consumers of medicine object because they are suffering. Health maintenance organizations object because they are paying for ineffective medicine. A new group of doctors will get excited when they see permanent resolutions of diseases without side effects. These are the doctors of tomorrow. These are the doctors that patients are demanding today.

Disease resistance requires a powerful healthiness that is beyond the normal training of medical doctors. The limited concept of "free from symptoms" can ignore imbalances that lead to disease. The benefits of super health include a full lifetime of wellness and energy.

Drugs and surgery have a valuable and important place in health care. But with many medical problems there is time to try gentler treatment options. Lifestyle changes are often the gentlest and most effective approach. First we can cover the basics: the right food, personal fitness, rest, and relaxation. Then we can move on to increasing our health to its full potential. This includes cleansing and strengthening any body systems that need help. We can remove stressors and toxins. We can aid the eliminative systems. We can make sure that nutrients are there when our bodies need them.

We all normally consume pounds of food and drink every day. While other factors are important, diet may be the single most important influence on our health. A natural diet is vital for perfect health and disease resistance. Americans are constantly tempted to eat damaging empty foods. What modern medicine often tries to do is to offset pounds of bad food with a few milligrams of chemicals. This can never work in the long run.

There are many alternative remedies that a conventional doctor may not know about or use. These are not just new drugs or procedures to be prescribed as any other medical therapy. There are philosophies behind each type of therapy. The mode of action with natural healing is rarely to attack germs or to manipulate chemicals within the body. Instead, natural healing supports our own healing power.

Our medical system is based upon drugs. Americans consume thousands of tons of pills every year. Over three billion prescriptions were filled in America in a recent year. Prescription drugs cause well over 100,000 deaths each year and millions of side effects are crippling Americans. Many of these side effects can be prevented when safer, natural techniques and remedies are utilized to their full potential. We can often avoid drugs by first trying helpful changes in our lifestyle, and then proceeding to utilize natural therapies. This book will help us to understand how to avoid disease and build a strong health.

Our medical professionals can also learn to take into account the tainted air, water, and food that are so common in our modern environment. It is easier to resist illness if we are not polluted by our surroundings.

The hospital is where we go to have our lives saved, yet it has also become a profit-oriented industry. Peace and dignity are difficult to achieve there. From a consumer's perspective, our hospitals can sometimes be scary places. This book will help you to find alternatives to hospitalization. If you must go, this book will give you a checklist for a safer and more pleasant stay in the hospital.

For the vast majority of health problems there is time to use gentler, safer, and more permanent approaches. Only after exhausting the natural solutions, or in an emergency, should we resort to chemical drugs and surgery. The good doctor's most important rule is "first of all, do no harm."

We need to heal medicine if it is to heal us. We need a new medicine that is based upon the strengths of both modern medicine and natural medicine. For maintaining health and for healing chronic diseases, natural medicine is often best. For emergency care and acute illness, modern medicine is best. Both approaches to health are good in their correct place. Together they form a complete health care system.

We can relearn how to become our own best doctor. We can learn to take responsibility for our own health. We can support a healthy life with sensible choices. It is not so difficult or complicated to create perfect health. Let me show you how.

PART I

HEALING
MEDICINE

Chapter 1

How We Heal

With a natural healing approach, the focus is on the person rather than on the disease. The method is to support the natural process of healing without interfering. This is a gentle, sensitive, yet powerful approach that takes into account the individuality of the person. Natural healing works on an infinitely finer scale than the scalpel.

Carefully supported natural healing can allow our bodies to heal on a cellular level. No surgical approach can do this. Natural treatments are based upon the accumulated experience of many generations. This experience is not only based upon science, it also is based on knowledge, wisdom, and common sense.

There are many diverse approaches possible in natural

healing. These approaches improve the patient's physical, emotional, and mental capacity to fight illness. Everything we do, our entire lifestyle and attitude, affects our health and our capacity to resist illness.

With natural therapies, bad side effects and treatment-caused illness are unusual. With natural healing we assist nature. These natural healing principles are the very ones that modern scientific medicine considers itself to have long ago outgrown. Hippocrates called the natural self-adjusting powers of the body the *physis*; this is the root of the word *physician*.[1] It is only by supporting the natural balance of the body that true healing can take place.

Natural healing does not generally need to identify or cure diseases. Natural healing eliminates diseases by cleansing and strengthening body systems to resist diseases. If we do what makes us healthy, health problems disappear. Health problems can generally be reversed by the same lifestyle changes that would have prevented them in the first place. For example, reducing meat intake not only prevents gout, but it cures it as well.

Some doctors may argue that you cannot prove scientifically how natural healing works. Let us suppose that we find a very ill person in a dark, dingy room all alone and without money or friends. Now let us suppose that this ill person is taken to a bright, cheerful home and cared for with love and great food. Let us imagine that this ill person starts getting some exercise and a new purpose in life. It is easy to imagine that this ill person might get well. So which thing "cured" him? No single change is solely responsible for the gain in health, yet this single "cure" is what scientists are looking for. This is why natural healing is often called holistic. Holistic refers to the whole person, including his or her environment.

Throughout the history of medicine there have been two

ways of thinking. The scientific medical way of thinking wants to prove theories. Nothing is called real unless you know exactly how it works. The other way of thinking, called *vitalism* or *empiricism*,[2] accepts as valid anything that has a long history of being safe, natural, and effective. These natural remedies are accepted even if no one knows how they work. Vitalist therapies include most natural therapies such as food therapies, medicinal plant therapies, traditional Chinese medicine, Ayurvedic healing, chiropractic therapy, homeopathy, massage therapies, and many others.

How Medicine Heals

Medical drug treatments provide a substitute for the healing processes of our bodies, often with costly, high-risk chemicals. These drugs either kill pathogenic germs, or they attempt to regulate our bodies' internal chemicals. Antibiotics act as a substitute for our immune system. Chemotherapy kills bad cells instead of our own immune system killing them. Synthetic steroids replace the hormones that we should be making. When histamine levels are too high, as in hay fever, doctors will block them with antihistamines. Insulin is given in an attempt to regulate our blood sugar levels. In each case a healthy body could do a better job than the chemical manipulation. In each case, our bodies are less able to do their job after the therapy.[3] There is no precedent in evolution for the introduction of these chemicals into the human body.

There is more to consider in revising medicine than the overuse of drugs. Medicine can also be a bit nearsighted when considering symptoms. It is vital to consider individual characteristics beyond just the immediate symptoms of the disease. The environment, lifestyle, diet, and fitness are the first places to look. Other areas of potential imbalances, such as body toxicity and mental attitude, must also be considered. Unfortunately, today's medicine often concentrates too much on the sickness and too little on the lifestyle factors that made the person sick. Treating just the symptoms results in short-term cures. A recurrence of the medical problem is all too common with a "symptom-treat" approach.

One way to look at how a modern medical doctor thinks is to compare a doctor's approach to that of a military commander. The uniforms of these medical generals are surgical masks or white lab coats with stethoscopes. The enemy is the disease. The disease is often considered separately and independently from the person. The doctor attacks the enemy inside the person. As in the military, direct action and attack are seen as necessary. While the doctor is focused on and attacking the disease, the patient seems almost incidental.

This type of medicine has a relationship with the disease more than with the person who has the disease. This type of doctor needs to be impersonal like a military officer. From the frontline skirmish in the emergency room to the big guns in intensive care, the similarities can be seen. If the person is hurt by the battle with the disease, well, side effects and treatment-caused illness are the risks of this type of war on disease. Where there is an acute need for lifesaving techniques these risks are acceptable and reasonable. On the other hand, with chronic disease and milder ailments these techniques can cause too much collateral damage when compared with gentler approaches.

How Nature Heals

A good doctor understands how nature heals and supports that healing. Doctors don't heal us; our bodies heal themselves. We can aid healing and recovery in many ways. We can remove impediments to the healing process. For instance, a hostile emotional environment might be suppressing immune function. We can increase the strength of the body and build powerful health. We can strengthen any of the systems within the body by removing stressors and toxins. We can aid the eliminative systems to clean up our internal environment and make sure that nutrients are there when our bodies need them.

Many people think that drugs and surgery can heal them. However, taking chemicals or getting a body part surgically removed does not always provide long-term healing. True healing needs to support the body's *own* intrinsic processes, and it involves eliminating the cause of the illness or injury so that it does not come back. On the other hand, some of the methods that medical science employs result in increased susceptibility to further problems.

One example of increased susceptibility happens after antibiotics are prescribed. The initial infection may well disappear. However, the antibiotics weaken our bodies in many ways. When our good bacteria are killed, this encourages yeast to grow out of proportion. Yeast infections are common after a round of antibiotics.[4] Normally our good bacteria help to keep yeast under control. By killing digestive bacteria, antibiotics also reduce nutrient absorption, including vitamin B12.[5]

The bacteria themselves are often made resistant to the antibiotic so that stronger antibiotics are needed the next time. Allergies can develop to antibiotics. Many people have experienced weakness and digestive discomfort as a result of antibiotic therapy. Most importantly, the patient is not strengthened to prevent the next occurrence of the infection.

Prednisone is another example of temporary healing. This synthetic steroid is often prescribed for inflammation. The inflammation typically is reduced right away. Did the drug heal you? Not really. The inflammation often comes back, worse than it was, after the drug is stopped. When our adrenal glands sense that there are enough synthetic steroids in our blood, they reduce their own output of hormones. When this continues for a long time the glands atrophy and can no longer produce enough hormones on their own.[6] This is the opposite of healing.

Medicine must become more resourceful and use different approaches to support the healing ability of our bodies. With an infection, we must find the causes of the weakness and susceptibility that let the infection happen. Perhaps we should get prescriptions for more rest, controlling the impact of stress, and some diet alterations instead of drugs. Many common culinary spices help keep certain infections away; garlic (*allium sativum*) is one good example.[7] Many vitamins are helpful in supporting our own anti-infection systems; ascorbated vitamin C is a good example.[8] These types of solutions will result in a strong, infection-free person instead of one who returns to the doctor over and over.

Natural healing is normally slower than chemical medicine. It takes time for our bodies to regain balance. In our society, people often demand the fast action of drugs. We must be aware that the slower approach of natural medicine is not only safer, but can result in permanent balance and healing. We often heal in waves with symptoms coming and going in cycles.

The best approach is to use drugs to adjust our internal chemicals only after these safer and more permanent approaches have been given a chance. If there is time to heal naturally, then this is the best way. With a problem like borderline high blood pressure, the natural approach makes more sense than dangerous chemicals. With acute problems like a heart attack, it is too late to employ natural techniques.

Balancing Health

One glance at an average person will reveal many ways that this person may be out of balance. In many cases the person is overweight; two-thirds of Americans are now overweight or obese. It is not uncommon to see people with depleted energy. Poor muscle tone, uncoordinated movements, and lack of balance are common. Thinning hair indicates circulatory problems. A ruddy complexion may indicate an overly fast metabolism, an alcoholic problem, or a volatile temper. Breath and body odor may indicate clogged eliminative channels. Perceptive doctors look at these indications of an out-of-balance person. It is not enough to focus only on specific lab reports that relate exclusively to the presenting symptom.

Instead of figuring out how to plan a chemical attack inside the person, we must find out how to balance a person's health. The goal is to balance health, not just to get rid of a specific symptom like pain. With balanced health, many health problems simply disappear. Creating a balanced health is quite different than fixing a malfunction in a mechanical subsystem of the body. The three most important ways to achieve balance are diet, activity/fitness, and stress control. Without considering these factors, good health is just a happy accident. Without good health a person will have many return visits to the medical center.

There are two approaches to balancing health that modern medicine often ignores. The first approach is to take a good look at the patient and see what imbalances are revealed. We are looking here for imbalances that forewarn us of an illness rather than an actual disease. The second approach to balancing health is to analyze the *lifestyle* for deficiencies or excesses. Then we must teach the patient about these potential causes of disease and their consequences. The patient may then choose to correct the imbalances or choose not to correct them.

Regardless of the reason for a specific visit, an observant doctor will notice, for example, if the patient has a lot of pimples. A few questions about fried food intake and other fatty excesses will normally reveal the cause. Pimples can also be caused by an imbalance in hormones. The patient needs to know that the pimples are only a visible "tip of the iceberg" and that other problems deeper inside the body are also happening. For instance, free radical damage from the rancid oils in fried foods can deplete antioxidants and damage arterial walls.[9] Obesity is another complication of excess rancid fatty acids. The powerful addiction to French fries, etc. will have to be offset by the powerful knowledge of the consequences of eating them.

This concept of balance goes beyond the usual concept of "good health." Medicine defines good health as freedom from the symptoms of disease.[10] However, optimum health is much more than that. Optimum health means that the patient's diet is balanced, the patient's activity and fitness program is progressing nicely, and that the patient's stress and relaxation programs are balanced. The limited concept of "free from symptoms" ignores the imbalances that cause disease.

Consider a person who spends eight hours a day behind a desk and another four hours in front of a TV. If there is little exercise and no other activity, the person cannot be in balance. There may not yet be symptoms of a specific disease. The imbalances from lack of muscle tone, lack of circulation, excess weight, poor digestion, and a host of other *hypokinetic* (low movement) problems are sure to cause problems later. The chronic diseases that modern medical science finds so hard to cure *can* be cured and prevented by a balanced lifestyle.

When a person combines the usual faults of a typical American lifestyle, the "diseases of civilization" are inevitable. Fast food combined with massive stress and inactivity is guaranteed to cause disease sooner or later. We are all learning that prevention is the best "cure" for chronic disease. While medical science is confused as to the cause of cancer and heart disease, the best doctors are helping their patients plan a balanced lifestyle to prevent these diseases. Lifestyle planning will also serve to reduce the risk of a recurrence of a disease.

We all know that our minds play an important role in influencing our health. Mental and emotional balances have a powerful impact on health and disease. Even the strictest scientists recognize the power of the placebo effect. Happy, productive people can overcome a host of adverse lifestyle influences. Depressed and angry people cannot be completely healthy, because our minds and emotions control our hormone systems directly. The switch between the sympathetic "fight or flight" and the parasympathetic "relax and repair" states is based largely upon our mental perceptions of danger or security. Make sure that you and your medical professionals don't ignore problems with stress, sleep, and relaxation as causes of chronic disease.

The most powerful way to balance health is to eat an excellent diet. We need more than the minimum requirements of synthetic nutrients. We need a balanced intake of fresh food. When doctors want to look deeper into the causes and cures for chronic diseases, they will look at the diet record of their patients. Much of the story of how they came to be sick and how they can recover is written upon the dinner plates of the patients.

Clean On the Inside

Americans are almost universally over-consumers of food. Because much of this food is empty of real nutrition,[11] many are overweight and hungry at the same time. Americans eat an alarming amount of sugar, chemicals, preservatives, toxins, pesticides, hormones, and other unnatural additives in their food. These toxins are often eaten with lots of white, fiber-deficient foods. This causes a clogging of the eliminative channels when these channels are needed most. Instead of clearing out the toxins, these toxins are concentrated and retained. We can improve modern medicine by introducing natural techniques to clean the eliminative channels. We feel better and look better when we are clean inside.

The eliminative channels are essential for health: the colon, the kidneys, the skin, and the lungs. The liver can also function in elimination by releasing bile from the gall bladder. In a heavily clogged system even the sinuses and the reproductive system can release toxins. Most of these eliminative organs are somewhat clogged in most Americans.

Healing traditions throughout the world and throughout time incorporate cleansing into their healing. One example is from Europe where they use the medicinal herbs burdock (*arctium lappa*) or dandelion (*taraxacum officinale*) in the spring to clear liver toxins. Naturopathic doctors systematically clear each of the eliminative channels. More importantly, these eliminative channels are kept open with the right food and health habits. American medicine has largely ignored keeping these clogged systems clean. The best doctors see the positive impact of gentle system cleansing on virtually all health problems.

A Systems Approach

In these days of increasingly focused specialization, larger pictures of health and disease get lost. When medicine has a goal of curing *and* preventing further disease, the systems approach makes sense. This systems approach is also something that we can do for ourselves. We have all inherited some stronger and some weaker body systems. When a disease is found to impact a body system the best course is to strengthen that system. Merely hiding the symptoms of a disease will allow other diseases to develop in a weakened body system. The lifestyle choices that may have caused the disease will continue to undermine the system.

Some of the more important body systems to consider include digestive, muscular, breathing, blood circulation, nervous, skin, kidneys, and the liver-gallbladder system. Other important body systems include hormonal, immune, joints, bones, lymphatic, reproductive, and the brain. Body systems all influence each other. When they are all working in harmony, we are healthy. Specific therapies may be needed for certain problems of a body system. However, general strengthening and cleansing of the systems involved always makes sense. Disease is just your body's way of pointing out that a system needs help.

If there are problems with digestion, for instance, we need to take a close look at the diet and stress patterns of the person. Foods or stresses that cause one digestive disease may well cause others. By cleansing and strengthening the system, the current disease will be reduced and future diseases will be prevented. When a drug is prescribed for a digestive disorder, the digestive system is not normally strengthened or cleansed. The only long-term cure for digestive woes is to eat a diet for which the digestion is designed. Whole grains, vegetables and roots, fruits, nuts, and seeds are foods to fuel digestive bliss. Meat, dairy products, white flour products, sugar, caffeine, and other processed foods can lead to digestive distress.

If there is a cramping muscle, a shortsighted approach is to simply prescribe antispasmodics. Muscle spasms occur when tight muscles get strained. However, these muscle strains will most likely happen again if the muscles are not stretched and strengthened. Daily stretching and toning of the muscles is the only long-term cure for muscle strains. A more effective approach will also train the patient to use his or her body so that muscles, tendons, and ligaments are not strained. Poor quality mattresses, fast, jerky lifting, and acidic wastes from meat eating all contribute to muscular problems. Hot baths, massage, hot packs, inversion, essential oils, and swimming can strengthen, stretch, and relax the muscular system.

If a person has breathing problems, modern medicine normally uses drugs to suppress the problem. Many breathing problems come from mucous congestion. The smart approach is to reduce mucus-thickening foods in the diet such as dairy products, eggs, and white flour. The medical approach to breathing problems often doesn't consider pesticides or chemicals in your air; it may not consider smog. Any approach to breathing problems that doesn't address the freshness of your air is missing an important factor. In winter in America, there is often very stale and polluted air in the home.[12] Workplace air should be considered as well. A holistic doctor will help you strengthen your lungs with breathing exercises, aromatic inhalations, expectorant medicinal plants, and good old fresh air. The advantage to this systems approach is that future problems are prevented as current problems are cured.

Our blood circulation system is powerfully affected by our food, our stress, and our exercise patterns. If your cholesterol is too high, the medical approach is to prescribe drugs. However, with any but the highest cholesterol levels there is time for gentler and more effective approaches. Our medical advisors can teach us that our bodies make enough cholesterol for our own needs. They can teach us that only animal products contain damaging cholesterol.

If you have high blood pressure, the medical approach is to prescribe drugs to lower it. This is another situation where there is often no emergency, so gentler, long-term approaches make sense. A good approach would be to set you up with a stress reduction program, a tailored fitness program, and a relaxation program. In addition to specific therapies, there are many general ways to strengthen our blood circulation system. Regular aerobic exercise, rebounding, vitamin E, hawthorne berries (*crataegus oxyacantha*), inversion, deep relaxation, natural diet, and massage all contribute to a trouble-free blood circulation system.

Nervous system disorders are normally treated with drugs. It is important to note that troublesome nerves may not be getting the nutrients that they need to function properly. It makes sense to look at what is fraying your nerves in the first place. We must not overlook things like excessive caffeine and fatigue that may be causing these nervous problems. No matter what drugs are given or what body part is cut out, these causes may remain. Without addressing the causes, it is very likely that a nervous problem will return or others will start. Specific natural therapies are available for specific nervous system problems.

There are many natural ways to benefit the whole nervous system. Although Americans get an overload of fats, essential fatty acids are almost universally low. Evening primrose oil (*oenothera biennis*), vitamin E, and high-quality organic, cold-pressed oils are helpful for nearly any nervous disorder. The elimination of bad oils in the diet can also help greatly. These bad oils include hydrogenated fats like margarine, rancid fats found in fried foods, and the engineered oils on supermarket shelves. Some of the other ways to avoid frayed nerves are taking naps, lessening driving stress, reducing media over-stimulation, lowering caffeine and sugar intake, and enjoying more love.

Our skin can be considered a body system. Our skin is constantly building new cells and pushing the older cells out. When these dead cells are not rubbed off, a host of skin problems arise, especially fungal problems. Brushing the skin, using a loofa in the shower, and wearing natural fiber clothes all contribute to healthy skin. Regular, limited exposure to sun is needed by skin, but erratic overexposure is very damaging. Regular sweating is needed to keep skin healthy.

Modern Americans rub an astonishing variety of chemicals on their skin. Many of these chemicals are absorbed into the bloodstream. Most fat-soluble chemicals and many water-soluble chemicals can be absorbed right through our skin.[13] Our digestive absorption is protected by the detoxifying efforts of our liver. However, chemicals absorbed through the skin can go directly into circulation. This can cause damage not only to the skin, but also to the kidneys, eyes, and other sensitive areas. If a lotion or oil is not pure enough to eat, it should not be applied to the skin. This certainly applies to any drugs that are absorbed as well. Using a systems approach, skin problems can become rare. It is when a skin problem does not respond to natural approaches that it is time to try drug approaches. Of course, we also need medical assistance for serious or dangerous skin problems.

When there is a problem with the kidneys or the urinary system, a systems approach also makes sense. Our kidneys are very dependent on the purity of our bloodstream. When meat is eaten in excess of our modest protein needs, it is burned as an energy source in our bodies. The metabolizing of meat leaves many acidic waste products in our blood stream such as uric acid, toxic amines, phenols, skatols, and pyruvic acid.[14] Our kidneys must filter these wastes out. With the excess of meat in most American diets, the kidney is simply not able to cope with these acids and wastes. We should not ignore this and allow problems to repeat over and over until surgery or dialysis is needed.

There are many simple ways to keep our kidneys healthy. Drinking plenty of purified water is a good start. Coffee and alcohol are two of the worst stressors for the kidneys. Regular sweating is very helpful to reduce the strain on the kidneys, especially in temperate or cold climates where sweating is less common. There are specific medicinal plant therapies for kidney stones, urinary tract infections, and other problems.

The key to a successful systems approach is to cleanse, nourish, and strengthen the whole system that has experienced a problem. We must find the lifestyle factors that have caused the problem and change them. This is the path to true healing. Prescription drugs and surgery may be needed, but they should only be used where lifestyle changes and gentler therapies have not completed the healing.

Chapter 2

Beyond Symptoms

The process of diagnosis is an integral part of modern medicine in America. Because treatment is determined by the diagnosis, diagnosis is one of the most important parts of the medical procedure. We need to find and understand the important clues as to what started the disease process. We need to take into account the vast differences between individuals and to consider the unique history of lifestyle and environmental factors. Doctors are trained to look for disease; they also need to be trained to build optimum health and to identify the root causes of disease.

A Deeper Diagnosis

The finest complete physical exam cannot pick up many serious health problems including imminent heart attacks, strokes, and aneurysms. Modern medicine is puzzled and regrets that these "accidents" befall their patients. However, these are not accidents. It takes many years of poor diet, stress, and poor fitness to produce an increased vulnerability to these chronic diseases. It is not hard to diagnose these vulnerabilities from the lifestyle. We have decades to predict and prevent disease and many other health problems. Even with a seemingly clean test panel, some patients are clearly at risk for certain diseases. If a person is highly stressed, eats lots of meat and dairy products, gets sporadic heavy exercise, and gets virtually no vitamin E, he or she can be diagnosed on this basis. If this person is over forty, there is a very high risk of heart disease.

Modern medicine is expert in and very effective at diagnosing and treating accidents. Doctors and hospitals are also very skilled at pulling people through a crisis resulting from chronic disease. It is too late to employ natural medicine when a stroke is happening. However, it is still important to employ the techniques of natural medicine after a stroke to decrease the risk of another stroke.

Today's medicine depends on experimental science for its understanding of disease, yet science can be unreliable when applied to a person, their inner systems, and their environment. Furthermore, science today is not always objective. Financial and political pressures sometimes mold the results of experiments and studies. While experimental science is idolized, empirical science is largely ignored.

Doctors are highly trained in the study of diseases. This training can be made more helpful if doctors can use natural healing methods in response to their scientific diagnoses whenever possible. Differentiating between diseases is a skill

How Does Your Doctor Rate On Diagnosis?

Does he give diagnoses gently and with optimism?
Does he just mask symptoms or does he cure causes?
Does he check your diet record for causes of disease?
Does he evaluate your fitness program?
Does he take into account individual differences?
Is he aware of environmental influences?
Does he look at emotional causes of disease?
Does he evaluate your stress profile?
Does he look at your nutritional supplements and spices?
Does he listen to his intuition—and to yours?
Does he rely exclusively on lab test results?
Does he use his eyes, nose, and hands to aid diagnosis?
Does he assume the worst and give "shotgun" medications?

of doctors. Treating the disease in a way that resolves it permanently and without damage is a skill of natural medicine. Doctors can work with natural practitioners, each helping in their own way. It is even better when a doctor understands both diagnosis and natural treatments.

Medical diagnosis has the potential to focus the doctor on the disease rather than on the person. The doctor can become immersed in considering thousands of diseases instead of the person in front of him.

Another way to improve diagnosis is to take a reasonable amount of time to come to a decision. Snap decisions are dramatic, but a more careful evaluation can save lives. It is wise for patients to ascertain that their hospital doctor is not exhausted. Exhaustion and time pressure can push even the best doctors to a hasty diagnosis. A hasty diagnosis can result in inappropriate drugs being administered, many of which have potent side effects.

Medical diagnostic tests can also result in incorrect diagnoses. Some lab tests are unreliable. Some of the tests themselves are dangerous and invasive so that the diagnostic procedure causes injury. Many lab tests are done unnecessarily. As patients, we can make sure that our tests are really necessary.

Hearing a diagnosis can sometimes be dangerous to your health. There is an intensification of stress when a diagnosis is made. This can impair the immune system when it is needed most. Some doctors will say, "You have breast cancer and your chances of living another five years is only five percent." This will shock the patient and suppress the immune system. Fear and uncertainty are not conducive to healing. Many doctors know this and choose to phrase the diagnosis in positive terms. A gentler doctor will say, "You have a serious problem. We can work together in many ways to reduce the risks, but breast cancer is always difficult." This gives a positive feeling that the patient can work with the doctor to reduce risks.

Because it is the patient's immune system that fights the cancer, it is best to keep it working. Our minds powerfully affect our immune system. Wise medical practitioners know this. The best presentation of a diagnosis allows us to know what we can do to resist the disease. It is also important that any diagnosis is presented in such a way that the patient can see how to avoid future bouts with the same illness.

Diagnosis also defines the incapacity of the patient. The diagnosis often makes the patient dependent on further medical findings. This can lead to enforced inactivity and concentration on the disease. People need to be productive within their capacity even while sick.

Medical diagnoses often ignore the root causes of the disease. Diagnosing the current disease without removing the causes can result in return visits to the doctor for similar problems. Let's look at some of the ways that doctors can make smarter diagnoses.

COFFEEDONUTITIS

It is not uncommon for a medical diagnosis to be couched in long, confusing Latin words. There may be a more productive way to present a diagnosis. A person may come to a doctor with sharp stomach pains that occur around ten-thirty in the morning. Some doctors might diagnose "gastroenteritis" (this means irritation of the stomach and intestines), and prescribe a chemical with the potential for many bad side effects. A deeper look at the problem might reveal that the patient eats donuts and coffee a couple of hours before each episode. What if a diagnosis of "coffeedonutitis" is made? With a diagnosis that indicates the cause of the problem, the cure is obvious and does not involve any potentially nasty side effects.

With a diagnosis of gastroenteritis and a chemical drug to offset the symptoms, the patient may be set up to experience side effects and continued problems. The side effects

Daily Diet Record

Name _____ Date _____

Please list all foods, snacks, and beverages. Estimate the
amount of each.

Breakfast

Midmorning

Lunch

Afternoon

Dinner

Evening

might cause nervousness, for example, which might then be treated with psychoactive drugs. This can lead to a downward spiral of health.

With a diagnosis of "coffeedonutitis," the cause of the problem can be addressed. In addition, there may be other effects from the coffee such as anxiety. The "side effects" of reducing coffee could be positive. Similarly, the donuts may be causing obesity or pimples. It is smarter to reduce consumption of donuts and coffee than to prescribe drugs in this case. It is clear that this approach is one that spirals health upward. Our medical professionals need to understand the health effects of different foods and common habits.

Unique Diagnosis

People are as different on the inside as they are on the outside. There is an incredible variation in structure and chemistry between people. Roger William's book, *Biochemical Individuality*,[1] gives excellent graphic examples. Bowels may be long and convoluted or short and simple. Hormones and immune systems vary greatly between different people. Blood vessels vary in size and elasticity. Some people have quick, sensitive nerves while others are relaxed. In light of these variations, different people need different treatments, even for the same symptoms.

Doctors do consider many variables in their differential diagnosis of disease. However, they are differentiating between which diseases the symptoms define. This is different than considering differences between people with the same symptoms. Different people with the exact same symptoms should get different treatments. Today's medicine often ignores individual differences between people. While the variation in disease is considered, the variation in people is not. Treatment works better when doctors learn more about the person in front of them rather than just concentrating on disease identification.

A health history is a useful tool to differentiate between diseases. However, without knowing the diet, fitness habits, lifestyle, and environmental influences, the history is incomplete. Unfortunately, it is not common for these factors to be taken into account, partly because it takes more time to analyze these lifestyle factors. Also, most doctors have not been trained to interpret these lifestyle factors. With time and training, we can find the primary causes of the disease. This is much better than just finding which symptoms to mask. The key here is to look at long-term improvement of the patient's health.

Extensive and expensive testing is often used to find out which disease is present. Interpretation of these test results often leads to disease names that sound like a medieval priest's Latin incantation. The patient is often befuddled and confused by this type of diagnosis. This does not help get at the root of the illness and is the opposite of teaching the patient to care for himself. What we need is to be taught how to take better care of ourselves.

Some people have large stomachs and some have small ones. Some people have too much stomach acid and some have too little. Some people have stomachs damaged by coffee and alcohol. Of course, the diet has a large influence on the function of the stomach. Stress plays a role in the function of the stomach. Yet, our medical system is set up to give each person the same drugs for the same stomach complaints. There must be more variation than just compensating for body weight.

TYPES OF INDIVIDUALS

Most traditional healing systems from around the world *do* take into account the individual. Classifications of individuals are essential in understanding the person, the causes of the disease, and the correct remedies. While none of these traditional systems exactly fit the medical needs of modern America, there is much to be learned from their attention to the individual. There are usually many possible remedies for any illness. When choosing between these remedies, it is important to consider individual differences. In this way, we get more effective remedies and balance the person as well.

In India, the Ayurvedic system has different remedies for the same condition depending on the constitution of the individual. If the person is *Pitta*, this means he or she tends to be too hot with a fast metabolism. An example of this would be a person with aggressive energy and a reddish complexion. This person might need a cooling, calming remedy. If a person is *Vata*, this means that the person is airy and leaning towards intellectualism. An example of a Vata person is a person with anxiety and a thin, light body. This person would benefit from eating grounding root vegetables and other strengthening foods. A *Kapha* person is watery and often overweight. Stimulating and diuretic actions would be balancing for this individual. Doesn't it make sense to tailor any remedy to the type of person?

Traditional Chinese Medicine has many ways of classifying both the individual and their syndromes. A yin person is thin and light, while a yang person is stronger and heavier. Diagnosis in Chinese Medicine is highly involved and takes into account many aspects of the individual person. A specific syndrome is identified and a remedy is tailored to the individual from the remedies for that syndrome. For example, one person with a cold may get a totally different remedy than another with the same symptoms. In America, our current medical system prescribes the exact same medication for the same symptoms regardless of the patient's characteristics.

The Classical Homeopathic system of medicine is elaborately tailored to the individual. Dozens or hundreds of questions are asked to get a complete picture of both the individual and the disease. The history of the disease is carefully noted. Attention is even paid to the time of day that the problem occurs.

In *Eclectic Herbology* the remedy is tailored to balance the person. While the main effect of the medicinal plant or formula is to help the disease or symptom, the remedy is also chosen to balance the person in many ways. If a person is too warm or too cool, the remedy is adjusted to balance this. If a person is too moist or dry, different remedies will be chosen. A sluggish person will get a different remedy for the same disease than a stimulated person. Some people could use a diuretic or laxative action. There are many remedies for any disease; tailoring them to the individual makes for more effective medicine and better health in the long run.

There are other factors used in diagnosis in other healing traditions. Smell is an important clue to many health problems. Some of the abilities of the nose are unmatched by the largest laboratories. Doctors around the world use their sense of smell. Many American doctors would consider it undignified to engage in the unscientific act of sniffing. Pulse diagnosis and tongue diagnosis are interesting diagnostic techniques of Chinese and Unani medicine. Doctors might be interested to learn the basics of these diagnostic techniques or refer them out as they would a lab test.

Intuition and instinct are used by healers worldwide. Unfortunately, medical schools train doctors to ignore these insights. Using only intuition is clearly not a whole system of diagnosis. And yet, any system of diagnosis that ignores the deeper wisdom of man is also not whole. A little common sense can help with any diagnosis.

Modern medicine is becoming informed as to how these excellent systems help find the correct remedy for the person, not just for the disease. This has been a deficiency in our present medical system of diagnosis that can be corrected.

Wrong Diagnosis

Eyes, fingers, brain, intuition, experience, noses, and ears can all assist in reaching a diagnosis. It is not enough to rely only on test results, especially if they contradict the human senses. Experienced doctors know that test results can be wrong. It takes time to get to know a person and to know what ails him.

A quick diagnosis without enough time spent to fully evaluate the individual leads to many mistakes. In one study, 104 patients were started on antibiotics for strep throat when only eight of them actually had strep throat.[2] We must not assume that antibiotics do not cause harm in the other ninety-six patients. This technique of assuming the most serious disease and dosing the patient with powerful drugs can be irresponsible.

Many people believe that the diagnoses of modern medicine are infallible. Nevertheless, diagnosis is a difficult and fallible process. In one study doctors were tested by having them look for lumps in silicone models of breasts. Even though they had time to look and feel carefully, and were aware of being tested, they missed the lumps fifty percent of the time.[3] In real women, this exam is even harder because breasts change over the month and vary greatly from one woman to another.

A common diagnostic procedure is the mammogram, which looks for breast lumps. Mammograms expose the woman to a high dose of x-rays, 250-1000 millirads per mammogram.[4] This is a great deal more than an average chest x-ray. In fact, only a few other x-ray procedures (such as the gastrointestinal series with barium) have higher exposure to x-rays.[5] Breasts are more easily damaged by radiation than most other body parts—in fact, one book finds that an astounding seventy-five percent of breast cancer is caused by x-rays.[6] Mammograms may not reduce the number of breast cancer deaths.[7] The real question is whether early detection of breast cancer saves more lives than are lost due to the increase in cancer as a result of this test.

Even when a mammogram reads negative, it may be wrong between five percent and sixty-nine percent of the time.[8] Because this uncertainty about the dangers of mammograms exists, it may be best to teach women to diagnose themselves for breast lumps. Women can get to know their own body and how it changes over their cycle. Women can do this self-exam much more often than they can go to a medical office. If a lump is found, then the woman can look for further information from a professional.

Diagnosis of underlying causes is harder with psychological problems. Even though psychiatrists are medical doctors, they often overlook the physical causes (like needed nutrients) of psychiatric problems when making their diagnosis. And primary care physicians make the wrong psychological diagnoses in many cases.[9]

Medical diagnoses often ignore the real causes of the problem. For instance, half of the one hundred million[10] yearly visits to emergency rooms are due to medication problems, street drugs, or alcohol abuse. Yet the diagnosis of alcohol or drug dependency is given in fewer than five percent of the cases.[11] We need to get at the root causes of the problems.

DIAGNOSIS AND RESPONSIBILITY

One of the reasons that modern medicine can fail to understand what their patients need is the factory approach to medicine. It is difficult for doctors to examine the patient and the lifestyle factors in twenty-two minutes, which was the average exam time in 1999.[12] Many hospitals lowered their routine pediatric exam time to ten minutes in 1992.[13] Routine exams make up five percent or about fifty billion dollars a year, of health spending.[14] Taking time to really get to know the diet, environment, fitness, and stresses of an individual would be necessary for a successful outcome. I would like to suggest some techniques to show how an efficient doctor of the future might handle many patients a day and still have long-term success.

In the clinic of the future, disease trends can be reversed in the individual patients. When an appointment is made, history forms can be mailed, faxed, or emailed to the patient a week or more in advance. During the next week the patient can fill out the diet and fitness forms in daily detail. The environmental questionnaire can detail sources of toxins and *carcinogens* (cancer-causing chemicals and hard radiation). Family, job, and personal stresses can be recorded on another form.

Computers are beginning to be able to read these forms and flag areas of concern for the doctor. Doctors using these techniques may need further training to know which of these factors are causing the health problems of the patient. We can look at the whole spectrum of health problems, not just the presenting symptoms. The diet record can be evaluated by computer for vitamins, minerals, complex carbohydrates, bad fats, and many other factors. Fitness records can be translated by computer to charts that display periods of aerobic exercise, strengthening, stretching, recreation, walking, and rebounding.

With the patient's help in filling out the health histories and the computer's help in printing a concise summary, the doctor of the future may be able to get much done in a short amount of time. Yet, time is still important. In a pediatric infant exam, for instance, there is too much to do to limit the exam to ten minutes. The doctor must take time to learn how the baby is sleeping and what the baby is eating. The doctor needs time to see if the baby is crawling, walking, or talking. Extra time is essential to spend on an infant exam to catch any irregularities early. An experienced doctor can do an excellent job if given enough time. Limiting a doctor to only a ten-minute exam is a dangerous insult to a sacred service. Average exam time for adults is about twenty minutes; however, two-thirds of medical exams are under fifteen minutes.[15]

The wise doctors of the future will de-emphasize germs and drugs. They will balance and correct the habits that cause problems or susceptibilities. These doctors will educate their patients so that the patients understand the source of their troubles. They will know that it is very important to explain in plain language how the needed changes will resolve the problem.

Chapter 3

Primary Prevention

True prevention, also called primary prevention, makes patients so healthy that they need doctors less and less. HMOs (Health Maintenance Organizations, like Kaiser) and insurance companies can save money if they increase their use of true prevention. True prevention teaches us to maintain healthy habits in food, environment, fitness, and stress. For impoverished people, primary prevention involves good nutrition, sanitation, clean water, and decent housing. Medical school curriculum includes less than two hours of instruction in these types of prevention.[1]

In three areas, HMOs can and do prevent further health declines. Sponsoring "stop smoking" programs is an excellent way to prevent disease. Counseling obese people on fitness and diet can also really help. Diabetics can learn how to eat to help control their blood sugar swings. The unique outlook of an HMO is that healthy people cost less in health care. This is the first time we have had such a powerful force to promote good health and prevention.

Unfortunately, the word prevention has been corrupted. The responsibility for prevention should be with each of us. Instead, modern medicine uses the word prevention without much participation in primary prevention. Regular physical exams do not prevent diseases; they detect diseases. Other screening programs also do not actually prevent disease.[2]

Health screening can give us false results that make us think we are sick when we are not. In the case of the tuberculin and other tests, dangerous drugs may be prescribed for people who do not need them. Health screening transforms public health clinics into referral machines for medical services and products while the need for true prevention goes unsatisfied.

Physical exams often do not prevent illness with our current medical system. When a problem is detected during a physical exam, this normally results in a drug being prescribed or surgery being performed. These medical procedures may mask the symptoms or temporarily remove them, but the factors that caused the disease may not get changed. Diet, lack of exercise, and unremitting stress are not commonly looked at in typical physical exams. The patient can end up with the side effects of the drugs or surgery plus symptoms when the disease returns, and it is likely that the disease will come back unless the causes of the disease are changed.

Prevention Is Better Than Cure

The idea that we can prevent disease through lifestyle changes is not popular with modern medicine. This idea is not popular with the patients of modern medicine either. We like to think that disease is just an accident. We like to think that we just happened to be standing in the wrong place and it "got" us. Our health professionals should assist us in learning which lifestyle mistakes cause which diseases. We must learn to take full responsibility for the choices we make that produce disease in us. The consequences of not doing so are all around us.

No experienced car owner would neglect to change the oil. Nor would anyone put anything in the gas tank but gas. We don't run our cars over top speed until they blow up. With cars, maintenance and prevention are only good sense. We don't normally believe that car problems are an accident. Properly maintained, cars last through the warranty period without problems in the majority of cases. If a mechanic merely fixed a car's problem without checking to see if the fluids and fuels were correct, if the mechanic did not look for pending problems and perform routine maintenance, these "accidents" would befall these cars much more frequently.

Some people never seem to get sick. Others get sick frequently. As long as our medical system is looking primarily at germs and genes, it will remain blind to the true causes of disease. It is not that germs don't exist or that they don't cause disease. It is that germs only cause problems for susceptible people. Bacteria and viruses remind us when we have weaknesses. Disease reminds us that we need to change our life. Medicine must learn to teach us what needs to be changed. When the changes are made, not only does the disease go away, but also, more importantly, it does not return.

There is one interesting thing about the changes needed to prevent illness. The changes that prevent one illness often have a preventive effect on other illnesses. In other words, the side effects are good. As body systems get stronger and cleaner, total health generally improves.

Health Maintenance Organizations (HMOs) are becoming a major factor in patient care in the second millennium in America. While their cost cutting strategies will cause much grief due to under-treatment of patients, some good may also come from HMO management. Since the financial mandate of the HMOs is to keep people healthy, many of the health-building strategies in this book will become desirable from a profit perspective. HMO doctors are struggling with patient care versus their own economic survival. In this book, they will find economical ways to create health instead of expensive ways to temporarily set disease back.

Our medical system needs to learn to analyze our lifestyle and habits and suggest changes that will prevent the type of problems that we are having. Some extra training may be required so that doctors can recommend the correct changes. A doctor with this training can put you on a path where your health starts to improve generally. This is a positive reinforcement where body systems come into balance and health improves. This is just the opposite of the health deterioration that so many patients now experience.

PREVENT AND TREAT THE COMMON COLD

The common cold is one example of a disease that is thought to be transmitted by germs. However, some people never get colds, even when exposed to them. Other people get colds even when they are not exposed to cold germs. Germs cause colds only when a person is weak, clogged up, and susceptible. It is easy to catch a cold. Just miss a lot of sleep, eat poorly, and get chilled a few times.

The accent should not be on curing the cold, but rather on preventing it in the first place. It will go away in a few days by itself. If we are strong enough to resist colds in the future, then colds will no longer be a problem. An informative health professional will explain exactly why a person is susceptible to colds. Then this professional can explain how to become immune to colds. Once the patient recovers from the cold, the patient can diminish the frequency of colds to zero. As health habits improve, the incidence of colds will diminish.

What are the mysterious miracles that prevent colds? Limiting mucus-thickening foods such as cheese, eggs, and milk is an excellent first step. Providing plenty of fresh fruits and vegetables will provide the needed nutrients and cleansing factors. Keeping white flour and sugar out of the diet as much as possible is very effective. Restful periods of time and good sleep are very helpful. Exercise is needed to cause sweating and purge toxins. These are general suggestions. A careful look at a diet and fitness record will reveal more causes of cold susceptibility. With these lifestyle changes, cold germs will "bounce off."

In order to treat colds, we must understand them. A cold is a cleansing process. It is best to work with the natural process of cleansing rather than working against cleansing. Decongestants work against this natural cleansing process. We are aided by the virus in cleaning out our sinuses, throat, and lungs. Colds go through several distinct stages and each needs a different kind of support.

In the initial stage there is a sore throat. Medical doctors often recommend over-the-counter painkillers or wrongfully prescribe antibiotics. Antibiotics are ineffective for a cold. The painkillers allow the patient to go to work or school instead of resting and healing. This can increase the risk of the cold worsening to flu, bronchitis, or pneumonia.

About Colds

Prevention: Eat lots of fresh fruits and vegetables, get enough exercise, get good sleep, and stay warm. Limit dairy products and white flour.

First stage, sore throat: Drink lots of soothing, hot tea. We use licorice root (*glycirrhiza glabra*) and raspberry leaves (*rubus idaeus*) with a squirt of echinacea (*echinacea angustifolia*) tincture. Rest and stay warm. We use 1000 mg doses of ascorbated vitamin C as well as topical applications of echinacea tincture mixed with propolis to the throat to numb, coat, and heal.

Second stage, mucous elimination: Let the mucus flow out and replace with plenty of hot tea and juices. Warmth and rest are needed.

Last stage, lung cleaning: Continue warmth and rest and soothing herb teas for the throat. Gentle plant antispasmodics will help with the coughing.

The correct treatment for this stage is rest, lots of water and juice, and plenty of warm medicinal herbal tea with soothing, pain-lessening, and antiviral properties. At the same time one thousand milligram doses of ascorbated vitamin C and applications of diluted echinacea tincture to the throat should be considered. This boosts the immune system and gives our bodies a head start on the road to completion of the cold. If this treatment does not reduce the pain enough, painkillers can be used.

The next stage involves cleansing the sinuses. Many over-the-counter cold medications dry up mucus. The normal medical routine is to try to stop this natural cleansing. This is not advisable because the mucous discharge is helping the body to clean itself out. At first the nose is stuffy. Aromatic steams and hot tea help get the mucus flow going. It is necessary to keep the patient warm and quietly entertained. The next stage is blowing the nose. *Demulcent* (internally soothing) medicinal plants in the hot tea, such as marshmallow root and licorice root, help keep the fluids flowing without irritation. We are supporting the body here instead of suppressing it. Again, what is most needed is rest.

The last stage is the cleansing of the throat and lungs. Warm clothes help the hot tea melt the congestion. The medicinal teas should be soothing internally with expectorant properties. The goal is to support the body in bringing up the mucus. In the later stages of coughing, there may be spasmodic coughing. Chamomile (*matricaria chamomilla*), valerian (*valeriana officinalis*), blue cohosh (*caulophyllum thalictroides*), and skullcap (*scutellaria lateriflora*) are medicinal plants that gently prevent spasms while allowing the expectorant process to continue. Lobelia (*lobelia inflata*) tincture was originally outlawed partly because of its incredibly effective and immediate antispasmodic effects on coughs.[3]

The final stage of an illness is convalescence. Convalescence involves gradually re-strengthening the person and the breathing system. We can wind up with a healthier and cleaner person at the end of the cold.

IMMUNIZATIONS

There are many factors that determine whether or not a person gets a disease. Housing, nutrition, environmental factors, fitness, stress levels, and many other factors determine the strength of the immune system. The initial strength of our immune systems is boosted by good nutrition before and during pregnancy as well as by breast-feeding.

Breast-feeding is a vital part of the development of the human immune system. All of the specific immunizations in the world cannot equal breast-feeding for reducing disease and strengthening the immune system.[4] The physical and emotional stress of formula feeding damages the immune system for life. Breast milk contains specific antibodies that the mother has developed. This passes on the mother's resistance to disease to the child. Baby food also plays an important role in the developing immune system. Over-processed empty baby food is no substitute for pureed fresh food. The lack of enzymes, fiber, vitamins, and minerals in over-processed food retards the development of the child's immune system. The presence of additives, pesticides, excess fats, salt, and sugar are also detrimental.

Our goal is to be immune from diseases. Specific immunizations like flu shots or polio vaccine are useful for people in poor health who have impaired immune systems. However, there are other ways to prevent disease. The healthy human immune system is incredibly powerful. We can mobilize millions of tiny warriors in a matter of hours. Attacks by virulent microbes on truly healthy people do not always result in illness. Legally required immunization vaccines have helped to stamp out some diseases. However, another way to prevent disease is to build the health and immune system of the person. If we are not stressed all of the time, if we eat fresh foods, if we exercise to maintain fitness, we can become largely immune to disease.

We must each carefully research and evaluate each vaccine and make an informed decision as to its utility and dangers. Flu shots are rarely effective because there are so many changing strains of flu. Ironically, flu shots often cause side effects similar to the flu. The polio vaccine is good for public health. However, for an individual child, the polio vaccine may risk as much disease as it prevents. Diphtheria has all but disappeared, but immunizations continue. In the rare outbreaks of diphtheria, the immunizations are proven to be unreliable in preventing the disease.[5] Cellular whooping cough vaccine is effective in only half of the recipients and the side effects can be terrible: high fevers and convulsions.[6] Since whooping cough is rare, the vaccine may be more dangerous than the disease.

The measles/mumps/rubella vaccine may increase a child's chances of brain inflammation and autism.[7] Measles vaccine is given to prevent measles encephalitis. In well-nourished children the incidence of measles encephalitis is extremely low. The sometimes-fatal side effects of the vaccine make the vaccine of doubtful benefit. The vaccine for rubella (German measles) also is of dubious safety due to the possible side effect of painful arthritis, which may last for months.[8]

Today, some immunizations may cause more harm than good. It is difficult to find information on the dangers of immunizations. Funding is lacking for studies that will decrease the vast profits from immunizations. We should each become informed and decide carefully for ourselves and for our family. State law requires children to get immunizations to attend school. Are these state laws there to protect our children or are some of them the result of pharmaceutical lobbying?

TAKE A NAP

In modern America, one of the most common causes of ill health is fatigue. The stressful and high-paced lifestyle continuously erodes our reserves of strength. Caffeine and freeways push Americans faster. Media bombardment seems continuous in a frantic effort to sell everything. Even on vacation, Americans seem to have too much to do.

One of my favorite teachers, Dr. Bernard Jensen, has a saying, "All sick people are tired people." Certainly, unremitting stress suppresses immune response. The solution will not make billions for a drug company. The cure will not keep clinics full. A great antidote for American life is a nap.

A nap is a time of an hour or two with peace and quiet, normally taken in a quiet, secure place. Noise, media, and phones should not intrude as this is the time to sink into a deep rest. Afternoon is a good time for most people, either by themselves or with lovers, children, or animals. The whole point of a nap is to rest peacefully without demands or interruption. In many countries of the world, a nap or siesta is a way of life.

Why is it that modern medical science cannot prescribe a nap? Even with obvious diseases like adrenal insufficiency and chronic fatigue syndrome this obvious cure is ignored. There is no pharmaceutical advertising money to promote naps. Yet this is a safe and natural treatment that can be suggested for many ills. Find out for yourself the healing power of the nap.

TAKE CARE OF YOURSELF

Modern medicine is not focused on building strong

health. Lifelong medical supervision is not intended to strengthen our health. In fact, many of the drug therapies degrade our overall health while helping a specific problem. We are browbeaten into thinking that we are medically incompetent. Sickness must not cease to become the concern of those who are sick. Certainly, the constant barrage of conflicting media stories on health is of little help.

The only solution is to take charge of our own health. Use self-awareness and self-discipline to control your life. Make informed changes in your own diet, exercise, and lifestyle. See how they affect your own health.

PART II

HOW WE GET SICK

Chapter 4

The Causes of Disease

Good health must be a priority. Many Americans make the decision to work too hard, too much, and too fast. We need to understand the need for rest. Even at play, Americans do everything hard and fast. We all need to see that unremitting stress and work are major causes of many of the chronic diseases. As our leading experts on health and disease, doctors can help teach us to lead healthy lives. Peace, quiet, and a loving, restful life are important for health and disease prevention. These are also some of the ways to get well.

In other countries many people know that relaxation and a slower pace of life are important. Health is our real wealth. In America, we are expected to "strip-mine" our health in the pursuit of success and money. Fast food is generally bad food. Taking the time to make good food from fresh produce replaces this cause of disease with a cause of health. Chronic fatigue and a lack of time also keep Americans from pursuing fitness. These are the true causes of disease. When people are optimally healthy, fit, relaxed, and nourished, they rarely get sick.

DOWNRIVER

There is a story about a town called Downriver. Long ago, the people in the town noticed an occasional person drowning in the river. The Mayor organized a boat patrol to pull the flailing swimmers out of the river. As time went on, more and more half-drowned people were pulled from the river. The good citizens of Downriver responded by buying more boats and ambulances to bring the people to the hospital. The doctors became expert at saving people and pumping the river water out of them. With much high tech equipment, and at a very high cost, many of the victims were saved. But no one ever looked upriver and asked how all those people got into the river.

This story is a good analogy to heart disease. Heart disease is the most expensive aspect of modern medicine. Cardiovascular disease is the leading killer of men and women in America; 958,000 people die of cardiovascular disease each year,[1] forty-one percent of all deaths.[2] As the death toll grows, technological medicine grows more elaborate and expensive. At $326 billion a year, cardiovascular disease is bankrupting America.[3] Each year, 600,000 people have heart operations.[4] Many of these operations are only of temporary benefit because the diet and lifestyle are not changed. Now medicine has clot-dissolving drugs that cost twenty-two hundred dollars per dose.[5] These very expensive drugs can be heroic, but this approach is wasteful and temporary.

Modern medicine does consider certain causes of disease. However, without looking at the environment or lifestyle of the patient, the evolution of the disease is not clear. The most important causes of disease in America are food, inactivity, stress, chemical pollution, and emotional factors. These factors create disease over years and decades. The only real cure of a disease involves changing these causes.

There is a fundamental difference between building strong health and temporarily masking symptoms. Building good health is just what our medical system needs to do. Building good health involves educating people about what they did to get the disease. It is when a patient is experiencing symptoms that the patient is most open to hearing solutions.

THE DEATH OF THE GERM THEORY

There is a myth, perpetuated by our medical system, that we "get" diseases, that disease is a random and anonymous curse. This is a fallacy that allows the victims to be exempted from responsibility for their condition. In truth, we earn many of our diseases. The primary cause of disease is not a random attack by bacteria or faulty genetics. Disease occurs most often when our lifestyle harbors dangerous habits. We can choose our food and activity levels. We can avoid stress and chemicals. We have much control over our own health. I have seen that optimally healthy people are seldom bothered by disease.

Blaming bacteria or viruses for disease ignores the most important factor: susceptibility. The healthy human body has a most impressive array of defenses against intruders. Did you ever wonder why one person gets a disease and many

people around that person do not get the disease? Susceptibility to disease is the key, not exposure to pathogens.

Our air is teeming with bacteria and viruses; our food
and water also can be. There is no escape from exposure,

Colon Cleansing Program

The first order of business is to halt the intake of clogging food. Clogging foods have little or no fiber and have
a slowing effect on digestion. Foods to reduce or eliminate: meat, chicken, cheese, milk, white flour products,
and candy. A gentle cleansing would be a 25% reduction. Taking psyllium (*plantago psyllium*) seeds or soaked
fenugreek seeds (*trigonella foenum-graecum*) will increase
your fiber intake.

Drink plenty of pure water and hot herbal teas. Dandelion root, licorice root, and fresh ginger (*zingiber officinale*)
root make a mild laxative tea (simmer for a while). Avoid
coffee and hard alcohol.

Laxative teas that cause cramping are to be avoided. Vegetable and fruit juices help – fresh made is best.

Each person needs different foods to get things moving
without excessive liquidity. Cooked beets are gentle and
effective. Soaked prunes are very gentle. Vegetables and
potatoes are perfect.

Sit-ups are very helpful because they stimulate the peristaltic motion of the intestines. Don't overdo it. Remember that walking or other activity is very helpful.

but there is escape from risk. A child doesn't get a cold from a friend; the child gets a cold from the child's susceptibility due to poor health habits. The antibiotics that children so often get for their cold not only don't cure the cold, they don't address the reasons for the cold. We need to find and fix the causes of children's poor health.

Of the one billion colds yearly in America, the average child gets five to eight colds per year.[6] Each time the child may be brought to a doctor and given antibiotics. This is not so good for the child. Doctors need to analyze why there is a recurring problem. The siblings of the child may "get" the cold from him. I submit that the health of the siblings is suffering from the same deficiencies or excesses as the first child. It is the susceptibility to disease that needs to be addressed. Germs alone are not capable of infecting many of the surrounding, healthier children.

Some great ways to prevent colds include more fresh fruits and vegetables, reduced dairy products, less sugar and white flour, less caffeine, enough sleep, a peaceful home life, and enough exercise. Children with these advantages don't get colds even if sneezed on.

Germs can even be seen in a positive light. They remind us when our reserves of strength are low. They motivate us to build strong health. They remind us to rest. After all, bacteria make up half of our 100 trillion cells.[7] We can live in peace with bacteria if we build a powerful immune system.

DIAGNOSING THE CAUSE OF THE DISEASE

A person may suffer from anxiety and nervousness. Typically, tranquilizers or other psychoactive drugs will be prescribed to mask the symptoms. It would be better if doctors could spend a little more time to see if excess caffeine, driving stress, or family pressures are causing the problem. This could result in a more permanent cure and the avoidance of chemical dependency or toxicity.

It is not so hard or time-consuming to determine the causes of disease. Analysis of a week's diet record and a week's exercise and activity record will reveal many of the clues. Questions about the home and workplace will also reveal causes of disease. Our medical system is not yet designed to look for these causes of disease.

ELIMINATE THE OBVIOUS

Clogging of our eliminative systems is one of the most important causes of disease in America. The colon is the likeliest suspect. With modern America's diet of fiber-free meals, poor elimination of food wastes is almost universal. Most natural healing traditions around the world include a periodic cleansing of the colon by eating (or not eating) certain foods and medicinal plants. Blood cleansers such as burdock root are used to periodically clear toxins from the blood stream. It is rare to find American doctors who include natural colon cleansing or blood cleansing programs.

The skin is arguably the largest organ. Our bodies need to eliminate salts and other wastes through sweat glands. Deodorants, clogging lotions or oils, synthetic clothes, and makeup are examples of products that prevent the skin from cleansing. Rough toweling, saunas, loofa scrubbing, and dry skin brushing are some examples of natural therapies that help the skin do its job.

Most Americans drink little pure water. They drink sodas and coffee, beer and wine, milk and juices. Any water they do drink is likely to be contaminated with chlorine, pesticides, and chlorine byproducts like trihalomethanes. How can we maintain healthy kidneys with this input?

The lungs and mucous linings of the respiratory tract are also important and are a much abused eliminative sys-

---

Foods that Speed Digestion

(Fastest)	Apples
Oatmeal with fruit	Eggplant
Stewed prunes or raisins	Cabbage
Cooked beets	Cherries
Avocadoes	Berries
Corn on the cob	Potatoes
Brown rice	String beans
Whole grains	Bell peppers
Bananas	Corn tortillas
Chayote	Beans
Papayas	Tomatoes
	(Less fast)

---

tem. The thickened mucus caused by dairy products and other foods hampers the flow of pollutants out of the lungs. Air pollution and exhaust, not to mention cigarettes, damage the cilia that move the mucus out. Deep breathing, aromatic steams, and reducing damaging foods are ways that we can influence this system.

One cleansing technique involves controlled fasting. Although our current medical system does not use fasting as a tool, it is used in many areas of the world. Fasting is a powerful cleansing technique. Fasting must be done carefully and with expert help. Normally, complete fasting is avoided.

Modified fasting involves systematically reducing food intake. It must be carefully tailored to the person. Sometimes it is done with fresh fruit, vegetable juices, and herbal teas. Other times, raw foods may be used. For some, fasting may

---

Foods that Slow Digestion

(Slow)	Fish
Flour tortillas	Chicken
Dry nuts	Meat
White rice	Milk
White noodles	Eggs
White bread	Cheese
Pastries	(Slowest)

---

just be a slight decrease in the heaviness of the diet. By decreasing the constant intake of excessively heavy food, our bodies can start to eliminate wastes and toxins. Once we have achieved the self-discipline to stop all foods, it becomes easier to control food addictions and cravings.

UNDERSTANDING GROWTHS

There are many types of growths. This section will discuss the type of growths that result from too much toxicity in our bodies. When our bodies cannot eliminate certain substances they wall them off inside a growth such as a cyst. Due to clogged eliminative channels, these substances may not be able to be disposed of immediately. Our bodies have no choice; the toxins cannot be tolerated nor eliminated.

Therefore, they are walled off. Some of the worst toxins include trans-fatty acids (margarine is one source), pesticides, chemical drugs, free radicals, and irritants.

The key to resolving this type of growth is to restore the functioning of the eliminative systems. Resolving happens when the body can absorb and eliminate the toxins, thus reducing the growth. The influx of toxins must also be reduced. With proper elimination and a reduced toxic load, our bodies can eliminate many growths. This results in a much better healing than the approach that medicine often applies to growths. It is naïve to think that just cutting out a growth will cure the patient. This does not clear the eliminative channels nor does it reduce the influx of more toxins. Another growth is very likely to occur under these conditions because the causes still remain.

Prostate cancer may also have accumulated toxins as an underlying cause. The prostate is at the base of the bladder and surrounded by the colon. When the colon has been filled with rapidly putrefying food and loaded with toxins for many years, some of the toxins leak over to the prostate. Drugs and toxins eliminated from the kidneys go right through the prostate. The prostate is in the "sump" of the body. Just as in colon cancer, the irritating toxins in contact with the prostate gland for years at a time promote the growth of cancer. Sitting down for prolonged periods and a lack of exercise also play key roles.

Today, half of all American men will develop prostate enlargement that will affect urination.[8] Prostate cancer occurs in twenty percent of American men with 34,000 dying from it every year.[9] Cutting out the prostate will relieve the problem, but the same chemicals and toxins continue to affect other parts of the body. Surgery, therefore, is just a temporary reprieve.

What needs to be done is to clean up the body. This

should be done before the prostate cancer has developed. Ideally, our health professionals could teach us how to clean our colons and how we should eat to keep them clean. The key is to reduce the intake of toxins and to start purifying at the first sign of prostate problems. Waiting for it to get so bad that surgery is needed is a mistake. Prostate surgery is the fourth most performed operation; in a recent year, 250,000 surgeries were done.[10] Side effects of this surgery can be severe, with incontinence and impotence being common.

Another approach to resolving growths is *autolysis*, which is the process of breaking down our worst cells and using the raw materials (amino acids) for new construction. If our protein intake is low, then we need to break down cells in our bodies to have the amino acids to make more protein. Our bodies have enough wisdom to break down the least valuable cells. Doctors should take a close look at the diet of anyone with tumor growth problems. Over-consumption of protein is a problem because it reduces or eliminates autolysis. In addition, the metabolic byproducts of excess proteins are toxic. A normal vegetarian diet can be high enough in protein to supply all needs and yet still low enough in protein to allow some autolysis.

There are also ways to help the skin to pass the toxic substances through, if a benign growth is near the skin. There are certain valuable oils; one example is castor oil (*ricinus communis*), which makes the skin more permeable. Castor oil is unique in its ability to soak through the skin and purify the lymph system. There are clays (French green clay is best) that powerfully draw toxins through the skin.[11] Green clay is strong enough to neutralize and draw out many venomous insect stings like beestings. Many medicinal plant preparations also aid in resolving growths. Hyssop (*hyssopus officinalis*), St. John's wort (*hypericum perforatum*), and chickweed (*stellaria media*) are examples of medicinal plants that aid in resolving growths.[12] These are gentle and permanent ways to resolve growths.

Chapter 5

Breaking the Cycle of Stress

One of the most important causes of disease in America is stress.[1] It is important that we give more consideration to stress as a cause of disease. As a result, treatments will become more effective, and stress will cause less disease. When doctors look at stress and other lifestyle causes of disease, they can suggest corrections. This will reduce the stress or the impact of the stress on their patients, which is better than managing the effects of stress with drugs.

It is ironic that medical contact can create more stress. The delivery of a bad diagnosis is a shock to the system. Just entering a hospital is stressful. Dealing with the medical bureaucracy can be frustrating and stressful. Going to the doctor's office should be a pleasant, informative, and health-building experience.

FIGHT AND FLIGHT

Our bodies and minds have two contrasting states: the "fight or flight" state, and what I like to call the "relax and repair" state. The "fight or flight" state is also known as sympathetic nervous system stimulation. Modern life in America is designed to constantly stimulate the adrenal glands. Television, driving, movies, caffeine, and competition push us into the "fight or flight" state. In contrast, the "relax and repair" mode of life is harder to achieve. Lack of time, interruptions, and urgent calls make quiet time all but unattainable.

Our bodies carry reserves including glycogen (stored blood sugar) and adrenal hormones to deal with emergencies. These reserves are commonly depleted in Americans. Adrenal depletion and deep fatigue are all too common. This deep fatigue, combined with the "jazzed-up" feeling of stimulation, is at the root of many diseases.

Originally, our bodies developed this "fight or flight" response to deal with emergencies like an attack by a saber-toothed tiger. The immune system is suppressed for the duration of the attack. Our bodies wisely decide to put all energies towards short-term survival. When one stays in this state continually, the immune system cannot function properly.[2] Many infections and other immune system problems are due to suppression of the immune system by stress.

Because this prehistoric saber-toothed tiger could wound us, our bodies learned to constrict the blood vessels to the skin to prevent excess bleeding. The constant state of readiness for action causes constant constriction of skin capillaries. This restricts the capacity of our blood system and raises blood pressure. This type of high blood pressure is called "essential hypertension," and modern medicine has not identified a cause. We are now learning that the cause of many circulatory disorders is unremitting stress. The routine use of chemical diuretics to lower blood pressure can have bad side effects and lead to a lifelong addiction to the medication. It is more effective and safer to educate patients to avoid stress problems than to use a pharmaceutical approach. There are many excellent natural alternatives including stress reduction programs, medicinal plants, exercise, biofeedback,[3] supplements, and relaxation programs. Diuretic blood pressure medication should only be used as a last resort or temporarily in emergencies.

The most effective approach is to prescribe the only effective cure for the diseases caused by stress—rest. When given a careful explanation of why rest is needed, the patient is more likely to follow the doctor's order. A nap is one of the most powerful healing modalities. Many Americans never seem to rest. Deep rest is disturbed by television, loud music, or even movies. Warm baths, quiet book reading (phone off), and naps help achieve deep rest. This is good medicine.

HURRY UP

Hurrying is at the root of many diseases. This pushy, "type A" behavior is often admired in American society. In some other countries there is a slower pace of life. Hurrying is an important cause of nervous diseases from anxiety to chronic fatigue syndrome. In the good old days, a doctor would recommend a long ocean voyage or a resort visit to get patients to slow down. Maybe today's rushed doctors could learn from their more relaxed counterparts of old. Hurrying is the cause of so many ills of today.

Weekly Stress Record

Name _____

Start date _____

Please list everything that increases or decreases your stress. Estimate the intensity of each: 1 to 10 for more stress, -1 to -10 for stress relieving.

Monday

Tuesday

Wednesday

Thursday

Friday

Saturday

Sunday

HAVE ANOTHER CUP OF COFFEE

One of the greatest stress intensifiers is caffeine. It is found in copious amounts in virtually all American diets: in coffee, tea, carbonated beverages, even in some whiskey. From cradle to grave Americans are accelerated by caffeine, often aided by excess sugar. An observant person can spot the rapidly vibrating foot or hand of the over-caffeinated person. Can caffeine consumption be at the root of many diseases? You bet it can, from the eczema sufferer to the nervous wreck. What about *un-prescribing* caffeine instead of prescribing Valium or another sedative? Modern medicine is learning to *un-prescribe* many different destructive lifestyle habits as an alternative to using drug-oriented approaches.

TELEPHONE STRAIN

Telephones have become so ubiquitous that many Americans do not realize their demands. Day and night we are required to be instantly awake and alert to answer a call in ten seconds. This limits our ability to gain deep rest and activate our immune system. Another potent stress on Americans is being on hold on the telephone. Increasingly, we are subjected to long holds, often with annoying sounds. This is enervating and exasperating. Pushing buttons in the frustrating phone mazes of the automated machines is another stress. It is wise to take these factors into account when diagnosing and treating diseases of the nervous system.

Road Rage

One of the most powerful stressors for Americans today is driving. City driving is a real test of a person's equanimity. The instantaneous response time needed to avoid potentially fatal accidents is one factor. Our nervous systems were not constructed for such extended, microsecond concentration.

Another factor is that it often appears that another person, wielding thousands of pounds of steel, might kill you. This often leads to fear, followed by anger. Many personal needs are impossible to fulfill while driving. Restroom, food, and eye breaks are not an option at sixty miles an hour. We may be immersed in a powerful magnetic field while driving which may also have bad physical effects.[4] These are powerful challenges to our nervous systems, psyche, and adrenal glands.

Bad News

"The News" also affects our stress levels. Many Americans wake up to the powerful combination of caffeine and news. Whether it is the newspaper, radio, the Internet, or television, the stress is real and contributes heavily to the day's intensity. From local murders and rapes to distant military atrocities, fear and the "fight or flight" reaction are awakened. When evaluating stress profiles, news blasts should be considered as a possible contributing cause of disease. Sometimes cutting back to only getting the news once a week can reduce nervous stress and tension significantly. A simple test is to take your own blood pressure and pulse upon arising in the morning. Take them again after half an hour of

What Stresses You Out?

Hurrying?
Too much coffee?
Telephone strain?
Road rage?
Bad news from media?
Television?
Inactivity?
Family stress or loneliness?
Environmental stress?
Computer burnout?
Noise stress?
Hurrying while eating?
Bathroom stress?
Money stress?
Performance stress?

caffeine and news. On another day try taking blood pressure and pulse after half an hour of non-stressful activity. We can make these changes in lifestyle to see if the changes can reduce stress diseases and empower our immune system.

TELEVISION TRAUMA

Some Americans spend many hours a day sitting in front of a television. This affects health profoundly. On the plus side, watching television can be a break from a busy day and a time of relaxation. However, relaxation is hard to find with modern television programming. It seems that every show or movie is trying to stimulate those tired adrenals. Constant noise, shootings, terrible family events, and much worse are Hollywood's solutions to keeping you tuned to a channel. Some television shows try to scare you and the fear fills your blood with stress hormones. These constant stress hormones without any physical activity to release them lead to stress diseases. The most common is high blood pressure.[5] The inactivity itself is very bad for health if it is carried on for three to eight hours or more a day. Couple this with the advertisements for disease-inducing food and you could define a whole new series of diseases from television watching.

How can we moderate the effects of television? One way to help reduce the stress effects of television is to put an exercise machine in front of it. This allows a more natural reaction to stress; the stress hormones, primarily cortisol and adrenaline, can be worked off. At the same time some much-needed exercise can be accomplished. Exercise can also be an alternative to health depleting food treats.

In a way, much of television could be labeled "junk food for the mind." Constant exposure to angry, violent, mean, and stupid television can seriously affect the mind and emotions. Women are often portrayed as having value only if they are young and pretty. Men are portrayed as violent and as objects to create wealth. Caring, nurturing, emotional maturing, and a host of other healthy feelings are virtually absent from much television programming.

SCHEDULING FITNESS

One of the most common causes of disease in America today is inactivity. Activity moves the blood, removes toxins through sweat, circulates the lymph fluids, and strengthens the muscles and the cardiovascular system. Aerobic exercise even gives us endorphins to make us happy. The benefits of fitness are too numerous to enumerate. It is important to consider activity levels when diagnosing a disease. Part of the treatment for many diseases can be an improvement in the fitness program.

Americans sit down too much. We sit in front of televisions or computers. We sit at work or at school. Activity is further cut down by driving, standing, and riding. Our bodies were designed for many hours of activity each day. We just aren't getting it unless we make it a priority. This inactivity causes a host of modern diseases, and it contributes to other diseases. From hyperactivity in children to stress in adults, movement is needed.

A fitness evaluation is an integral part of an extended diagnosis. At least one week of fitness and activity should be evaluated. With a correct interpretation of the exercise record, incremental changes can be suggested to improve fitness. The relationship between inactivity and disease will become clearer with a fitness record. The effects of exercise on mood, muscles, and energy are dramatic.

There is no person who could not benefit from improved fitness. There is no disease that cannot be helped by appropriate changes in a fitness program. Your health professional can explain how each recommended exercise helps to keep illness or injury from returning. For example, many cases of constipation could be aided by abdominal exercise. This stimulates the peristaltic action of the intestines and aids in elimination. Certainly, other ways of relieving constipation should be used concurrently.

Preventive fitness will become more common as modern medicine recognizes its value. A person may come to a doctor with a sore back. The doctor may prescribe antispasmodics or drugs for inflammation. The doctor may

Weekly Fitness Record

Name _____

Start date_____

Please list all activities that make you more fit. Please note duration and intensity (1 to 10).

Monday

Tuesday

Wednesday

Thursday

Friday

Saturday

Sunday

tell this person to be careful lifting for a time. We can do even more by realizing that the same back problems tend to happen again. By keeping the back toned and limber with exercises, this person can prevent further back problems. Training in how to lift and move heavy objects is another key to prevention. Strengthening the abdominal muscles can balance back muscles and help to improve posture. We must learn how to avoid a string of identical back problems. This often involves looking at the work and home environment for back-stressing activities and back-stressing furniture.

There are many different types of fitness activities. An ideal fitness program will include most of them. These days we hear about aerobics and strengthening as the most popular forms of exercise. These are two excellent and necessary forms of exercise, but they do not encompass all of the needs of the human body for exercise. Breathing and stretching exercises are examples of other exercise needs. Yoga is a perfect blend of breathing and stretching. Yoga also helps with stress control. Regular stretching will prevent many injuries to muscles, tendons, and ligaments.

Inversion (hanging upside down or lying on a slant) is beneficial to the circulation, posture, eyes, and brain.[6] Inversion helps reverse many of the effects of gravity such as wrinkles and hair loss. Many of the sagging areas that we associate with aging can be reversed with a reversal of gravity. It is important to start with a moderate slant. A padded board leaning on the seat of a couch or chair might be a good start (some people use an ironing board). One can progress over time to hanging with gravity boots, if desired. It is recommended that a health professional certify your health for hanging upside down. Inversion can help with spinal disk problems. A few minutes of slanting will allow more circulation to heal the compressed disks than a whole day of standing or sitting. Additionally, climbing and hanging by the arms are excellent techniques for achieving better posture and giving room for the lungs and abdominal organs to work.

Rebounding (bouncing on a tiny trampoline) is excellent for circulating fluids and for coordination. Circulation of fluids is needed to deliver nutrients to areas of poor circulation. Rebounding also helps to clear toxins. Our lymph system is dependent on activity to move the lymph fluid. Rebounding helps move this lymph fluid.[7] There is a period of weightlessness during each bounce. This time of weight-

> *"Activity creates energy;*
>
> *inactivity breeds fatigue."*
>
> **Dr. Robert K. M. Cooper**

lessness is valuable for allowing the spine to elongate and decompress. While younger people can bounce, older people will find benefit even from bouncing their legs while sitting down. As with all exercise, start with a limited time and intensity and work slowly toward your goals.

Walking in the open air is a gentle stress reliever and a good counterpoint to our stressful society. Recreational exercise provides another human need—fun. For meek or fearful people, martial arts build confidence and strengthen bodies. Swimming is a wonderful exercise. One of the finest exercises is a light toning and working of all of the joints. Warm-ups from ballet, martial arts, and other sports give protection from tight tendons, shortened ligaments, and pulled muscles.

Fitness programs should vary for different people at different times. Sudden, unaccustomed exercise can be dangerous. Even though exercise is powerful medicine, it can hurt as much as help if done incorrectly. The age and fitness level of the patient must be carefully considered. Gradual building up to good shape is the key.

I challenge doctors to find exercise solutions for their patients. The side effects are positive. Not only can the current problem be prevented from recurring, but also many other problems that would have developed will not. Better fitness will also make you feel better.

FAMILY STRESS AND LONELINESS

In Hawaii they have a traditional healer who heals, not the person, but the family. Interpersonal stresses in a family can cause much stress and unhappiness. When people do not have a happy, welcoming, and relaxing home, they do not get the rest needed to heal. Acrimony between parents and children, siblings, or spouses can be the most important cause of many diseases.[8] People are sometimes driven to destructive health habits by family or roommates. Prescription medications are not the answer. Understanding the causes of disease and curing them will enable a long-term cure.

Another cause of disease is loneliness. Americans today are very isolated at work and at home. Unlike most of the world, many American adults and children sleep alone in an empty room. We spend very little time with people. Americans spend most of their time with machines: computers, televisions, lawnmowers, dishwashers, and so on. This lone-liness often leads to depression. Abandonment, alienation, frustration, and isolation are causes of depression. There are many excellent alternatives to prescribing Prozac, Zoloft, or Paxil. There are real causes of diseases, especially depression. Our health professionals can help us to learn what causes our diseases and how to prevent them.

Environmental Stress

The environmental causes of disease are very important and often overlooked. It is sometimes obvious that a hyper-active (Attention Deficit Disorder) child is triggered by food dyes, sugar, caffeine, or MSG (monosodium glutamate).[9] It is counterproductive to give the child a drug to counteract the food chemicals. The child gets both the side effects of the drug and the chemical reaction from the food additives. We can see from the diet record what the child is reacting to and suggest removing it from his or her diet. This way the side effects of both the food additives and the drugs can be avoided.

Our supermarket foods are loaded with pesticides, hor-mones, nitrates, and a host of other unnatural pollutants.[10] Our lives are often affected by cellular phones, electrical wires, microwaves, and even irradiated food.[11] Our water is often polluted with chlorine, bromine, trihalomethanes, lead, copper, mercury, pesticides, Giardia, and bacteria.[12] In mod-ern America, these potential causes of disease need to be taken into account during a diagnosis. Be sure to look at any job-related toxic problems as well.

Many of these environmental problems do not lead to an instant, noticeable disease. Instead, many of these envi-ronmental assaults take years or decades to contribute to cancer, lung disease, and the host of other chronic diseases of today. We must not discount environmental stresses simply because they produce no immediate disease.

Other common environmental stresses that can contribute to diseases include computer burnout, noise stress, hurrying while eating, bathroom stress, money stress, and performance stress.

The important point in this section is that diseases have causes. For too long we have allowed and even demanded that our medical system use drugs to hide our symptoms while ignoring the deeper causes of disease. This must stop. Informed consumers of medicine will demand this because their suffering continues. HMOs will demand this because they are paying for temporary results. A new group of doctors will get excited when they see a permanent resolution of diseases without side effects. These are the doctors of the future. These are the doctors who will be in great demand.

EFFECTS OF CAFFEINE

Caffeine can be a factor in many diseases, especially in stressed-out America. Caffeine works like most stimulants. It stimulates the "fight or flight" sympathetic nervous system. This simulates an emergency in the body. The immune system is given lowest priority. The skin capillaries are restricted to prevent blood loss in this simulation of an emergency. Blood sugar is released from stores to fight the unreal emergency. The nervous system and mind are especially stimulated. Eyesight is better; muscles are stronger. What could be wrong with all of this?

Blood sugar swings, hypoglycemia (low blood sugar), and diabetes are all impacted by caffeine. We keep a reserve of stored blood sugar, glucose, in our bodies. The storage is in the form of glycogen. You may think of glycogen as a little suitcase full of blood sugar in storage. Much of the glycogen is stored in the liver. More glycogen is stored in muscles for instant energy. When caffeine simulates an emergency situation, this stored blood sugar is released. This is one of the main reasons that the caffeine makes you feel so good. But this storage is there for a reason. When you need to call on your reserves of strength for a *real* emergency, they are not there.

Most caffeine users know that the stimulating part of the drug only lasts a while. Then the blood sugar goes down lower than normal. Blood pressure also subsides. The supercharged feeling goes away and is replaced with fatigue and irritability. Energy producing cofactors are used up, and the mind is depressed. We should consider caffeine use as a contributing factor in chronic fatigue syndrome and depression. Additionally, much mental instability is caused or exaggerated by caffeine. The initial blast of blood sugar also stresses out the pancreas as it tries to put the unneeded blood sugar back into storage. Along with the constant assaults of excess dietary sugar, this caffeine-released sugar causes diabetes after years of pancreatic stress.

The constant suppression of the immune system by caffeine is also responsible for disease. While caffeine does not cause infections by itself, it does keep the immune system inactive by stimulating the sympathetic nervous system. We all need constant policing of our bodies to prevent cells from spreading cancer. If we keep our immune system "switched off" every day, then our immune system cannot do its job.

Caffeine is also addictive. The energetic high is very attractive. To those who are depleted and exhausted it seems a necessity. When the three-hour high is worn off, there is an intense physical craving for more caffeine. In the morning, a caffeine enthusiast must have coffee to start the day. Most

Americans would no more consider giving up caffeine than giving up breathing. The coffee break is a staple of industry. Giving up caffeine often means days of headaches and fatigue. During this period the body rebuilds the depleted reserves of strength. The key to good health is to rest when tired. Caffeine allows us to hide our fatigue rather than rest. Caffeine is like having a credit card of energy. It is all too attractive to "overspend" and come up short later.

Another effect of caffeine is to stimulate energy production without providing the cofactors needed in energy production. In this sense it is like white flour and sugar. Energy is produced and the vitamins and mineral cofactors are used up, but no nutrient cofactors are provided. Couple this with the vitamin and mineral deficient white flour diet of most Americans and the production of energy aerobically is difficult. Fat burning becomes impossible as well.

It is not so much caffeine itself, but rather the constant, unremitting use of it that depletes health. When simulated emergencies occur every day, they deplete reserves of health. There is caffeine in many popular foods and drinks. From carbonated beverages to whiskey, Americans are inundated with caffeine. While parents are appalled by cocaine, speed, crack, and Benzedrine use by children, they may be unaware that their refrigerators are loaded with caffeine. The effects of caffeine are somewhat less dramatic than the effects of these other stimulants, but the health-damaging effects are very similar. This includes both psychological and physical effects.

HIGH BLOOD PRESSURE

In modern America we must become more aware of the relationship between caffeine, stress, and high blood pressure. Imagine for a moment that our bodies are like a city. Imagine that the water supply in the city is similar to the blood supply in our bodies. If the water supply is at a good pressure and then all of the faucets are turned off, what happens? The pressure goes up. This is exactly what happens when the "fight or flight" syndrome is triggered by caffeine or stress in our bodies. Our bodies are designed to close off the capillaries in case of an emergency to prevent blood loss from broken skin. When the caffeine emergency is declared too often, the volume of blood vessels becomes too small for the blood—raising pressure. In addition, the "fight or flight" reflex also directly raises blood pressure. Medical science calls this most common type of high blood pressure "essential hypertension" because a single specific cause has not been identified.

Just going into a doctor's office or hospital can raise your blood pressure. If your blood pressure is over the exact number that the chart decrees, you will most likely be given antihypertensive drugs. A large number of Americans, sixty million, have high blood pressure;[13] three quarters of these are on medication. Over sixty drugs have been developed to control blood pressure. These work on suppressing the symptoms of the problem rather than curing it. The most annoying side effect of these drugs may be loss of sexual desire.

There are dozens of safe, proven natural remedies for high blood pressure. If the blood pressure is not dangerously high, why not try these first along with a stress reduction and relaxation program? One example of a natural method of blood pressure control is called biofeedback. Biofeedback training is very effective in self-control of high blood pressure.[14] With thermal biofeedback training, you learn to let your fingers warm up with a sensitive thermal display. Fingers get warmer when you open the capillaries. Therefore, you are really learning to lower your blood pressure.

The causes of high blood pressure are obvious and preventable: stress, caffeine, bad fats, lack of exercise, and a constant state of "fight or flight." These factors constrict the blood vessels and increase blood pressure. Nature intended the "fight or flight" reaction to be invoked only occasionally. In a dangerous situation, the body would constrict the peripheral capillaries to prevent blood loss during a fight. From coffee and traffic, to stressed out work and power lunches, the blood vessels rarely get to relax.

DEALING WITH STRESS

Stress is a reality for most people in America. The best way to deal with stress is with a two-fold approach. The first part of this approach is to minimize the impact of the stress in the first place. This is the *Stress Control Program*. The second part is to relax and de-stress the person. This is the *Relaxation Program*. Doctors can use a stress record to see when the stress occurs. The stress record is simply a form that the patient uses to write down exactly when and where stress occurs. Normally, the patient records the stress record for at least a week. An electronic organizer or date book also provides many clues to stressors. Once areas of stress have been identified, programs can be developed to minimize the impact of each stress on the health of the person. While it is often difficult to change the situations where the person is stressed, it may be possible for the person to react differently in these situations.

For example, if a person is stressed out by waiting, techniques may be taught to minimize the stress of waiting. Reading a book, doing fingernails, using headphones with music, quiet meditation, or solving mind problems can be substituted for blood pressure-raising frustration.

Another common stressor is driving. Instead of getting mad every time someone drives dangerously or cuts you off, try counting how many times you encounter a bad driving move and rating them. Learn that your reactions to bad driving are in your own control. If people are the cause of the stress an assertiveness training course may bring some relief. The point is to identify the stress and stop it from hurting your health. Any effective medical system will have programs worked out and available to patients for each common type of stress. Health professionals can then monitor the stress until the patient can control it.

In modern life in America some stress is bound to be unavoidable. This is the time to learn more about relaxation techniques. Exercise is the best way to counter stress.[15] In particular, aerobic exercise is an excellent way to burn the stress hormones out of your blood. Talking over stressful situations with family or friends is another way to relax. Having a supportive family helps. Relaxation training is a way to completely relax your body in just a few minutes. With relaxation training or progressive relaxation, you take charge and dynamically cause relaxation.

RELAXATION TRAINING

For many people relaxation is elusive. Busy Americans do not have time to wait for relaxation to settle in naturally. Relaxation training was developed to empower people to relax quickly and on demand.[16] It is easy to feel like you have had a good nap after only five minutes of trained relaxation. Take control of your relaxation.

Find a comfortable spot where you will not be disturbed. It is best to lie down, but any comfortable position will work. A soft couch with pillows and subdued lighting is best. One can achieve deep relaxation even on cold concrete. Needless to say, this technique is also great for falling asleep.

Deep, regular breathing is the key. To take a truly deep breath, start by filling the lungs, continue to fill the stomach area, and finish by topping up the shoulder area. A good deep breath should take ten to fifteen seconds. To start off, take four deep breaths. While slowly taking the first breath, visualize yourself as totally secure. With the second breath, imagine that your whole body is warm. With the third breath, experience a heaviness of your body and a feeling that you are sinking deeper into whatever you are lying on. With the fourth breath, feel the breath as energy moving through your whole body as if it were a hollow tube and without resistance.

Now you can apply these four breaths to each part of your body. You can start with the feet. During a long, slow breath, imagine that you are secure from interruption or harm. With the second breath, visualize warmth in your feet. This visualization can open the capillaries of the skin to lower blood pressure. With the third breath, feel your feet get heavier until they seem to sink down and mold themselves to the surface. With the fourth breath, feel the surge of enriching oxygen move to fill the feet as if they were a hollow tube. Repeat the four breaths until the feet are warm, heavy, and open.

For each of the areas of your body, repeat the four breaths: security, warmth, heaviness, and openness. The security breath is important to activate the 'relax and repair' mode of your nervous system. It also activates your immune system. As you proceed to your ankles, extend the warmth, heaviness, and openness to your feet. Next the lower legs are relaxed with the relaxation extending to the toes. Continue with the knees, thighs, and pelvic area. Take an extra set of breaths to consolidate the deep relaxation in your lower body.

By now you will be getting better at having your body follow your thoughts. Continue with the stomach area, the lungs, the shoulders, the arms, and the hands. Continue with four slow breaths with a clear image during each breath. Next, let your face and head relax. To finish, experience your whole body as warm, heavy, and open. Feel your breath move through you, right down to your toes. During this restful time, think only harmonious thoughts and leave any difficult thoughts to be handled by your refreshed and relaxed self after this session.

The whole relaxation session can last from five to fifteen minutes and feel like an hour-long nap. One variation on this technique is to tighten the muscles in each area of the body and then release the tension to promote relaxation. This is the way Progressive Relaxation works. This tightening may make it easier for you to focus on each area. Feel free to come up with variations that work for you.

These techniques are much faster and more effective than just waiting for relaxation to occur. Naps or siestas are great ways to drop off the day's stresses. Hobbies or pets can be very stress relieving as well. There are many more techniques to relieve stress. Doctors can become more effective by using these techniques with their patients.

Chapter 6

Wholistic Food

We all normally consume pounds of food and drink every day. This food has a profound effect on our health. While other factors are important, diet is usually the single most important influence on our health. What modern medicine often tries to do is to offset hundreds of grams of bad and depleted food with a few milligrams of chemicals. This is difficult to do. Natural remedies also have a hard time reversing the effects of a bad diet.

What is a bad diet? What is a good diet? This all depends on whom you ask. It seems that whatever we ate in our childhood often appears to be the best and only diet. People are almost always addicted to their own way of eating. It is a very opinionated subject. It is true that we humans can eat many different foods. What I would like to focus on is which foods are best for health. The further we deviate from a "healthy" diet, the further we deviate from health and into disease.

Assuming that we know what a "best diet" is for a person at a particular time, how do we go about convincing that person to change? This is a challenge for any health professional who must know exactly why certain dietary mistakes cause certain diseases. Even more important, they must be able to explain this to the patient.

Doctors sometimes tell their patients to avoid certain foods. One heart attack victim said that his doctor told him to give up "everything that tasted good." People need to continue eating the correct amount of protein, fats, and carbohydrates after a diet change. Patients can be instructed on how to substitute better foods for foods that destroy health. In addition, there are many superfoods that build health in a variety of ways. One effective solution is to make a list of what the health advisor and patient consider bad foods. Make another list of foods that are health building. Have the patient eliminate one food from the bad list and add one food from the good list every week (or month). Sometimes patients are instructed to eliminate meat. This is not going to make much of a positive change if the patient just eats cheese, white flour, eggs, and processed food. Patients need to be informed as to which foods are health building as well as which foods are health destroying. Organic produce is the healthiest type of food.

Our dietary needs vary with age, climate, work and play, and many other factors. As we gradually change our diets, our dietary needs change, too. One example of this change is when we reduce meat and dairy products in our diet. After a time, we are then able to digest other foods much more efficiently because the digestive organs are less clogged up and coated.[1] Diet should be looked at as constantly evolving. We are each different with our own unique needs within the possibilities of digestion and metabolism. The differences in stomach size and shape, acid content, bowel length, metabolism, and many other factors make dietary change a very personal process.[2] However, even though we are all different, there are no humans with a carnivore's digestion.

There is a transition from a "normal" American diet to a diet more suited to our bodies. Many types of health professionals could benefit from further training in how to make this transition. Make sure that you choose a doctor or other health professional who knows how to guide you into a better diet. The changes must be gradual enough to avoid excessive cleansing reactions. A first step is often the reduction of meat in the diet. Other foods must be carefully chosen to compensate for the lack of stomach-satisfying meat.[3] A bowel-cleansing program can be employed to help eliminate the residues of meat digestion. Increased exercise and toning of the abdominal muscles can also aid this elimination. Your health professional must be personally familiar with these dietary changes for effective counsel. We need more attention from our medical system on how to make changes from 'normal' diets to healthy diets.

In this chapter, we will investigate the natural foods that humans and their evolutionary ancestors have been eating for millions of years. Only in the last few thousand years has technology enabled man to catch, cut up, and cook meat in any quantity. However, our digestive and metabolic systems have not changed. A few thousand years is too short a time for major evolutionary changes to occur in man. We have not developed the ability to deal with the excess protein and fat that are so abundant in meat. This excess protein and fat from meat are major contributors to many of the epidemic chronic diseases of today. Without meat and dairy products in the diet, arthritis, heart and circulatory diseases, cancer, and gout would not be major problems for vast millions of Americans. Other changes can reduce the prevalence of these epidemics, but reducing meat intake can help immensely.

Experimentation is one of the best ways to teach the changes in health that diet can bring. Personal experience is a powerful teacher. It also puts to rest all of the conflicting rhetoric on diet. One easy experiment is to eliminate all dairy products from the diet for a few weeks. Many people find that their mucous discharge is no longer present. Coughing, nose blowing, and postnasal drip seem to go away. It may not be so immediate, though, as discharge may go on for a while (sometimes years) after the dietary changes because the body must clean up the mess. After the dairy products have been absent for a while, eating a dairy product will result in obvious symptoms of mucous congestion. Yet, without this experiment, many people will go through their lives without knowing the cause of their health burdens.

Many people experience intense cravings for a rejected food as their body eliminates the residues.[4] The cause of these cravings needs to be explained. It helps to know that the cravings will recede over time. People sometimes confuse these withdrawal cravings for a real need for the food.

In most traditional systems of healing, food is the first medicine to be discussed. In Ayurvedic medicine the spices in food play an essential role in health and disease.[5] In Chinese medicine the effects of food are carefully accounted for.

Modern medical doctors receive little training in medical school regarding healthy eating.[6] They do learn a few therapeutic diets such as diets for diabetics, gout, weight reduction, and cholesterol reduction. These diets are not optimally healthy diets, however, partly because they are high in fat and rely on refined grains. When medical professionals need information about food they often turn to nutritionists.

Some of the nutritionist's books must have been funded by grants from the same food companies that bring you white flour, white sugar, and white grease. Nutritionist courses are often limited because they look only at what enters a person's mouth, ignoring the effects of soil, growth, processing, and storage on the food. Nutritionist courses also normally focus only on nutrients in food and often ignore damaging components such as pesticides and nitrates. This is outmoded thinking; we are developing new knowledge about the effects of modern food technology on human health and our well-being.[7] Many nutritionists do go on to learn more about natural healthy diets.

THE PERFECT DIET

Like other animals, humans have the ability to properly digest and metabolize only certain foods. Each animal has a diet that seems perfect for it. Humans also have an optimal diet. We can deduce the optimal diet by comparing humans to other animals. The proper diet for an animal is based upon logic. What people think is the right diet for humans is too often based upon irrational reasons or what tastes good to them. This is why I would like to look at what other animals eat—animals that are similar to humans. We can eat almost any food that we can swallow, but which foods are the healthiest ones?

It is clear that the healthiest foods must be natural foods that humans have been eating for a long, long time, not just in the recent technological past. We know that human teeth and hands have not changed significantly from the hominids (our direct ancestors) of three million years ago.[8] However, human diet has slowly changed over the past few thousand years.

More recently, in the last one hundred years, our diet has undergone extreme change with the advent of modern technology. Oils and grains have become refined. Food additives like nitrates in meat are now common. Mankind has shown a tremendous ability to adapt to these new foods, but only with a huge cost in sublethal (and lethal) breakdowns. Most of the supermarket foods today are vastly different from anything that the human body is designed to eat. This improper eating has caused the "diseases of civilization." Cancer, diabetes, prostatitis, emphysema, arthritis, hemorrhoids, heart and circulatory disease, and a host of other ills plague those who eat unnatural and processed food. The incidence of these diseases in those who eat natural diets is vastly lower.[9]

Some have advanced the theory that our gene pool can change because people die off from these "diseases of civilization." Some people think that humans have altered in the past few thousand years to be able to eat processed foods and not be damaged by them. This is not true as deaths are normally long after reproduction, so our gene pool is not altered. Also, it takes a long time for evolution to change a body. Once a small change occurs, it may take thousands of years to move this change through a population.

It is just not conceivable that today's humans could mutate to be able to eat meat or processed foods in this short of a time without increasing the grave risk of chronic disease. It would take millions of years for our genes to randomly alter to reduce our digestive length from thirty feet to twelve feet—allowing us to eat rapidly putrefying foods like meat. Twelve feet is about the length of a digestive tract for a carnivorous cat that is the weight of a man. It has already taken a million years for humans just to make small changes in face and body structure.[10] Our whole metabolism would need to alter as well. It is just as unlikely that humans will evolve into animals that can thrive on white flour, sugar, and pro-

Is Man a Carnivore?

Carnivore	Man
Claws	no
Swiveling ears	no
Dagger canines	no
Scissor incisors	no
Thin tooth enamel	no
Short digestive tract	no
Small liver	no
Speed	no
Fur	no
Close up vision	no
Track by smell	no

cessed foods. Eating foods that build health makes more sense than damaging our health with foods that are wrong for us.

ARE HUMANS CARNIVORES?

There is a spectrum of difference between an animal that is a perfect carnivore and one that is a perfect vegetarian. As we examine each part of a human, we see that we are far from being a carnivore and are, in fact, vegetarian animals.

Many people claim that humans are omnivores. This is not true in that we are not designed to eat many foods that other omnivores eat. Other animals classified as omnivores do not resemble man. Omnivorous mammals are timber wolves, foxes, jackals, coyotes, deer mice, rat opossums, and grizzly bears. These animals are naturally equipped to catch and

> *"Nothing will benefit human health and increase chances for survival of life on earth as much as the evolution to a vegetarian diet."*
> *Albert Einstein*

eat meat; humans are not. As we will see, humans are not naturally equipped to catch, butcher, chew, digest, metabolize, or excrete meat.[11]

There is a branch of science that studies the habits of man before historical records existed. Paleoanthropology bases its findings on the left over teeth and bones of early humans and their predecessors. The diet of humans is very hard to study from only bones and teeth. Prior to the Second World War, anthropologists thought man to be primarily vegetarian with the occasional opportunistic inclusion of meat. Because of the limited ability of man to catch, kill, and butcher meat, opportunities for meat eating were rare in early man. Because of food poisoning diseases such as *Salmonella, botulism, ptomaine, campylobacterosis, toxoplasma,* and *trichinosis,* eating previously killed animals could be deadly for man (prior to refrigeration and preservatives). Even with all of the technological methods of today, there are over 9,000 food poisoning deaths in America every year from eating meat. One hundred million pounds of meat are recalled each year because of contamination.[12]

Because of the horrors of the Second World War, paleoanthropologists looked for an excuse for man to be so brutal. They were convinced for two or three decades that man was a "hunter-killer."[13] This theory was debunked in the 1970s, and man went back to being described as primarily a vegetarian.[14] Unfortunately, many of the "baby boomers" were taught this incorrect myth and refused to reconsider. We will now look at the ways in which man differs from any of the "hunter-killer" animals.

Man has had the technology to catch, skin, cut up, and cook meat only in the last few thousand years. Prior to that meat was scarce or nonexistent in the diet. Before guns, meat was too hard to get to be a large or reliable part of the diet—despite ego-boosting myths to the contrary. Let us put aside our cultural and family bias for a minute and look at human food as we would look at any other animal's food.

Our fingernails are totally wrong for a carnivore. Carnivorous mammals (like cats) have retractable sharp pointed nails. We have flat nails that are unsuited for preying on an animal or for butchery.[15] You will see nails like ours on animals that are pure vegetarians. Gorillas have very similar nails, and they are pure vegetarians.[16] Gorillas and humans are close enough on the evolutionary tree to have similar blood proteins.[17]

Our ears are unsuited to hunting animals. Carnivores have ears that swivel to track prey, and our ears are much less sensitive than those of the carnivores. Carnivores have tough fur to protect them from struggling prey. Our skin is too fragile to resist the teeth, claws, and beaks of captured animals. Predatory animals normally have camouflage to help them hide from prey. Humans are un-camouflaged because fruits, grains, and vegetables have no eyes. Carnivorous animals have no sweat glands in their fur. These animals hunt at night and rest in the shade in the day. Humans, horses, and other vegetarian animals have sweat glands in their skin. Humans are primates, and the higher primates are very largely vegetarian.[18]

Our teeth are also not suited to biting through fur and hide or eating raw meat. Remember that we are looking at what the body is designed for, not what a body can do with technology. Carnivores have dagger-like canines to cut through hide and rip up flesh. We have some of the smallest, flattest canine teeth of all primates.[19] Other primates have larger canine teeth than humans. This helps them to eat tougher, more fibrous fruit and vegetables.[20] Carnivores also have scissor-like incisors. Man does not. In fact, our canines and incisors have slowly shrunk over the millennia to allow the side-to-side chewing action that is needed for chewing complex carbohydrates.[21] We have many molars to grind up grains and vegetables; carnivorous animals do not have molars. Our molars have the thick enamel characteristic of vegetarians.[22] Only strict grain eaters like cows have thicker enamel on their molars. Carnivores do not have this thick enamel on their teeth. Animals with teeth like ours have a diet of vegetables, fruits, grains, beans, nuts, and seeds.

Our digestive system is perfectly designed to get all of the nutrition out of starchy foods. Only vegetarian animals have this ability. We can secrete a digestive enzyme, *ptyalin*, in our mouths to predigest starches. Carnivores do not secrete ptyalin, but have stomach acids ten times stronger to kill bacteria and digest animal parts. Our intestines extract every iota of food value from starchy foods. With our thirty-foot intestines, we find that rapidly putrefying foods like meat, dairy products, and eggs slowly pollute our system.[23] We also have a large liver that is characteristic of herbivores. Herbivores need much larger livers to detoxify the toxins that plants use to defend themselves. Carnivores have much smaller livers. In addition, all carnivores synthesize vitamin

C in their livers. Humans don't synthesize vitamin C because we are designed to eat fruit and vegetables every day.[24]

Another characteristic of carnivores is that they can catch other animals. Man did not evolve with a rifle growing out of his hands. Naked in the wild, humans are not able to catch or kill other animals with any ease or reliability. We do not have the great bursts of speed that are common to all predators. Having two feet makes us slower and less maneuverable than practically any other animal. If humans were to catch a rooster, cow, or pig, they would be more likely to get hurt than to kill the animal. Many people have unrealistic delusions about being tougher than any animal. However, Darwin, the father of evolution, has written that early humans were fruit and vegetable eaters and that our form and anatomy have not changed throughout history. The great Swedish scientist whose classification of animals and plants is still used, Carl Linnaeus, states, "Man's structure, external and internal, compared with that of the other animals, shows that fruit and succulent vegetables constitute his natural food."[25]

The eyes of predators are also different. Their eyes detect motion better, but are not as good as human eyes in detecting colors. Humans see color very well. This helps us choose the ripest fruits and the best vegetables. Even our minds may have evolved to keep track of when and where fruit trees will ripen. Advertisers use pictures of ripe fruits and juicy vegetables to attract buyers. Pictures of ripped open animals are not attractive food packaging to most people. Our eyes are attracted to fields of grain and the colors of produce. Predators' eyes have very good close-up vision while we have better far vision. We tend to move away from something wriggling in a bush. Predators' eyes see wriggling in bushes as an opportunity. Predators have a much more acute sense of smell than we humans do. They are able to track prey by smell. Humans are incapable of this both because our noses are less sensitive and because our noses are not positioned near the ground.

Without cultural bias, we are clearly evolved to eat a nonmeat diet of grains, beans, fruit, nuts, vegetables, and roots. This is the natural, optimal diet for the human animal. The only question is how far we can pollute the correct diet before our health starts to fail.

TRACKING DIETARY NEEDS

If you go to a veterinary doctor with a sick animal, one of the first questions that he or she will ask you is about the diet of the animal. However, it is not normal in modern medicine to review diet records of people. A normal medical education does not include the analysis of diets.[26] Because illness is largely perceived as being caused by viruses and bacteria or accidents, the effects of diet on disease are frequently underestimated.

In my analysis of diet records, I have found that many diets analyzed were low in vitamin E and the B-vitamins. Trace minerals were often low in the diets analyzed. Vitamin C was also usually low. Essential fatty acids are virtually nonexistent in typical American diets. These days a diet record can be fed into a computer and an analysis of nutrients quickly printed.[27] Doctors can use this technique to diagnose deficiencies. They will quickly become convinced of the relationship between poor nutrition and disease.

Our bodies need vitamins and minerals as cofactors in the efficient charging of the cell's power battery, adenosine triphosphate (ATP). This ATP is like a rechargeable battery within the cell that is used for powering all of the cell's activities including muscle contractions. Without the right vitamins, food substances, and minerals, we produce only a small fraction of the energy stored in glucose (blood sugar). Vitamin B2, vitamin B3, and iron are examples of coenzymes needed to produce energy aerobically.[28] With the proper co-factors present, we can produce the full thirty-eight ATP's of energy stored in the glucose. However, we can only pro-duce two ATP's of energy from a molecule of glucose with-out these cofactors.[29] The more efficient method is called aerobic energy production because we are able to burn the fuel, glucose, with oxygen. This is a cleaner way to produce energy as well. The inefficient anaerobic (without oxygen) cycle also leads to waste products such as lactic acid being dumped into the blood.[30]

Without these vitamins, minerals, and some carbohy-drates, our cells are unable to turn fat into glucose (blood sugar). If even one of the vitamins or minerals is missing, the aerobic *Krebs cycle* cannot burn the fat.[31] The fat goes back into storage in our body rather than being burned. This is clear evidence that obesity is more than a genetic flaw; obesity is primarily a diet problem. When these factors are not taken into account, we have little success with fatigue and obesity problems. Adequate vitamins and minerals can increase energy efficiency by eighteen times. Our health care providers must learn that certain supplemental vitamins are essential when the diet does not provide enough nutrition.

Doctors who check diet records find that Americans are not getting enough nutrition for disease-resistance or opti-mum health. The daily amounts of vitamins and minerals recommended by the government are just enough to barely keep a healthy young person from developing signs of defi-ciency. The amounts of some of these nutrients are far short of ideal. In addition, it is difficult for Americans to get their nutrition from foods that are picked unripe from soils de-pleted in trace minerals. After refrigeration, processing, cooking, and storing, the foods do not have much left except carbohydrates, protein, and fat.[32]

Americans need extra nutrition because of pollution and stress.[33] Coffee, smog, driving stress, chemicals, rancid fried fats, and a host of other unhealthy influences create a need for more vitamins and minerals. Vitamins A, C, and E are known as antioxidant vitamins and are depleted by many of these factors. Therefore, between depleted foods and increased needs, Americans need either a super high quality diet or supplemental vitamins and minerals. I think we need both.

Epidemiologists have amassed some data on which diseases are related to which diets. Their research does indicate that eating meat and dairy products leads to many of the prevalent diseases of today.

BAD FOOD

What we are *not* getting in the diet may not play as large a role in health and disease as the wrong things that we *are* getting in the diet. Unfortunately, nutritionists are trained only to look at nutrients. We must not ignore food processing and contamination. Most meat and dairy products come from cows fed crops grown with pesticides.[34] These pesticides not only get into meat and dairy products, but a process known as *bioaccumulation* concentrates some of them. Bioaccumulation happens when an animal's cells store more and more of the pesticides from their food. Bioaccumulation normally increases the concentration of a pesticide by ten to one hundred times—sometimes as much as five hundred thousand times.[35] Then the pesticides are bioaccumulated and concentrated in the people who eat these foods. Fruits, vegetables, grains, and many other foods are contaminated by pesticides in America.[36] The organophosphate pesticides can create havoc with our nervous systems.[37] Organochlorine pesticides get into fat cells and promote cancer.[38] Organic food is a better choice.

When diagnosing diseases, pesticides should be considered as a possible contributing cause. There are many pollutants in American meat. Synthetic growth hormones are added to ninety percent of commercial beef.[39] These include cancer-causing synthetic chemical hormones such as estradiol, progesterone, and testosterone.[40] Antibiotic residues in meat cause resistant bacteria and encourage yeast infections in people. Nitrites are abundant in commercial meats in America. They are what preserve the red color of meat. They are converted into nitrosamines in the stomach and cause cancer.[41] Vitamin C can stop this conversion in the stomach.[42] It has also been found that nitrites themselves cause cancer without conversion into nitrosamines.[43]

For many years now many of the dairy cows in the United States have been injected with a genetically modified hormone, recombinant bovine growth hormone (rbGH). Because milk is mixed from many dairies, it is hard to find commercial milk in the United States that does not have this artificial hormone. Milk treated with rbGH may also contain higher antibiotic residues because these cows get more udder infections. Other countries such as Japan and those in the European Union refuse to accept this milk as safe. Human safety tests are sorely lacking for milk contaminated with this hormone. Another concern is that the genetically modified hormone raises the levels of another hormone in cows that may increase cancer susceptibility. This hormone (insulin-like growth factor-1) may greatly increase cancer risk for people who use these dairy products, especially breast and prostate cancer.[44] Organic milk and organic dairy products are free of these manufactured hormones and their associated problems.

The extra protein in meat and dairy products also damages health and causes illness. When we eat more protein than we need, the extra protein must be burned for energy. Our bodies have no storage system for extra protein. Burning protein for energy causes acidic wastes such as urea to build up in our blood.[45] This damages our livers and kidneys and causes fatigue.[46] These acidic wastes play a major role in producing arthritis and gout.[47] Excess protein also leaches calcium out of the body, contributing heavily to osteoporosis.[48] By keeping our diet low in protein, we can allow our bodies to use the wisdom of autolysis. In autolysis, our bodies take the weakest cells and the worst cells and break them up to use their amino acids to make new protein. When there is a glut of protein all of the time, this process cannot occur. Autolysis is one of the ways that our bodies destroy cancerous cells.

The extra fat in meat and dairy products also causes well-known and well-documented health destroying effects. We each manufacture enough cholesterol in our bodies to satisfy our needs. We do not ever need to eat any cholesterol from animal products, but when we do, we can damage our arteries and heart. The extra fats in these foods cause a host of diseases such as cancer, heart disease, and obesity. We do not catch these diseases from germs. We "catch" them from our food. Medical science recognizes that the consumption of animal products contributes to cancer, heart disease, and obesity.

WHY ORGANIC FOOD IS BETTER

Because diet is so important to disease resistance and health, we need to know which foods are better and which ones are worse. Because of the shortsighted greed of the food industry, food has lost much of its value. In the short run, it is cheaper to grow food with synthetic fertilizer and pesticides. This is a shortsighted approach because the bugs develop resistance and the soil becomes worse and worse. America tried to help the world grow more food by using chemicals and machinery. The result has been depleted soil, depleted food, and depleted health.[49]

Synthetic fertilizer is a mixture of nitrogen, phosphorus, potassium, and sometimes a few other minerals. It lacks all of the rest of the seventy-two minerals used by the human body. Every year the plants take out as much as they can get of dozens of minerals from the soil and every year the soil is fertilized with nitrogen, phosphorus, and potassium. After a few years there are almost no trace minerals left in the soil. If the plants do not get a mineral, then we do not get it from the plant. Thirty-two states are deficient in zinc in the agricultural soil.[50] Among its many uses in our bodies, zinc is needed by our immune system.

Besides the deficiency of minerals that synthetic fertilizers bring, there is another problem. The plants grow very quickly and very big. The plants are very weak and watery compared to organic produce. The complex of healthy organisms and bacteria that thrive in healthy soil are killed by industrial mono-cropping agribusiness techniques. The fruits and vegetables do look good, but they have little flavor or smell. It takes very little taste testing to be able to tell an organic apple. It smells and tastes like an apple, while the synthetically fertilized one has little smell or flavor.

Then there are the pesticides. By 1969 there were 900 basic chemical pesticides made into over 60,000 formulations.[51] Over half a million tons of pesticides are applied each year to our food.[52] Many doctors wrongly believe that pesticides are harmless when used on food crops. The truth is that most pesticides are dangerous to humans as well as to pests. One large class of pesticides is called the organophosphates. They work by incapacitating enzymes that exist in our nerve synapses. Without these enzymes, our nerves keep firing. The neurotransmitters that transmit nerve impulses in the millionth-of-an-inch gap between nerves need to be created and destroyed almost instantly. These pesticides cause a host of nerve problems from trembling to spasms to respiratory failure. These chemicals were developed as nerve gas agents by the Germans to be used on humans in war.[53]

There are many other classes of pesticides used on our food crops. They are all dangerous in their own way. Most of these pesticides are tested by big labs that have a financial incentive to approve these chemicals as safe. Some of the worst cases of testing fraud are associated with pesticide testing. Because these chemicals have not been properly tested, it is more important than ever to examine the pesticide intake of patients to see if pesticides are causing disease, especially in liver problems, spasmodic nerve problems, or cancer.

The pesticides from food production get into our bodies in two different ways. One way is from the residue on and in the food itself. Pesticides are often applied in a base of oil that resists washing off by rain or in a sink. Some farmers use pesticides in the soil so that the pesticides are drawn inside the fruit to attack insects. This is common with citrus crops. On many crops, farmers use a broad spectrum of pesticides. One study showed that thirteen different pesticides are used on lettuce;[54] this is not an unusual number of pesticides for a vegetable. If you are near a farm, you may be exposed to over-spray or windblown dust laden with poison.

Another way we are exposed to pesticides is when they get into our water supply. A tremendous amount of propaganda is used to convince us that pesticides are safe and do not ever get into our water. If you want to know about the safety of a pesticide, just look it up in Medline, a computerized database of medical articles (*www.pesticide.org/factsheets.html* is even better). You will quickly learn that there is no such thing as a safe pesticide.

If you are curious as to how much pesticide is getting into your drinking water, a water testing company can test it quite inexpensively. We can find and eliminate these causes of disease and instead build health by eating organic food. Please don't ignore these potent causes of disease and poor nutrition from eating commercially grown food.

Organic food is not allowed to be genetically modified. Genetically modified foods have not been proven safe and are not accepted in many parts of the world such as Europe. Most soy products in the United States come from genetically modified seeds—about eighty percent. These artificial soy products may have different nutrient levels such as lowered protein levels.[55] They may be contaminated with toxins. Cotton oil, canola oil, and corn, as well as Hawaiian papaya, are also commonly genetically modified. There are many documented cases of profit-oriented industry tampering with the safety testing of genetically modified food and drugs.[56] Safety from genetic modifications is another benefit of organic food.

UNDERSTANDING CULINARY SPICES

Garlic, ginger, basil (*ocimum basilicum*), thyme, cayenne, and most of the other culinary spices are actually medicinal plants. Although they may be partially inactivated by cooking, they can exert powerful influences on our health. Using spices in cooking is a pleasant and convenient way to take the medicinal herbs. Because they are taken in some quantity, they may have strong effects.

These cooking herbs can be used to balance a person in many ways. One person may have a sluggish metabolism. For this person, cayenne would probably taste good and be balancing. Cayenne speeds up the metabolism and warms the body. Another person may have chronic infection problems. For this person, garlic in the food can be a healthy alternative to periodic assaults of chemical antibiotics. Unlike chemical antibiotics, garlic, echinacea, and larch (*larix occidentalis*) keep your own immune system strong.

Some doctors take into account which spices you use on your food. In fact, these spices can sometimes cause imbalances. If a hot, speedy person uses a lot of cayenne or ginger, it can cause an aggravation of these characteristics. Even common salt or pepper can cause problems. Ulcers may be caused or aggravated by mustard or horseradish. On the other hand, mucous congestion might be reduced by these same two spices. The spices need to be tailored to the person.

In Ayurvedic medicine, culinary spices are the primary way to get medicinal herbs into people. The Ayurvedic doctors study each person to find which herbs are needed or balancing. They also check the diet and the current spices used by the person. From this and the health history, an Ayurvedic doctor can tailor spice intake recommendations. Sometimes the only cure needed is a few spices in the diet. Unlike Western medicine, the cost is small and the side effects are good.

When the right spices are used, a person feels better right away. Even the cooking smell is a clue when it smells just right. When you smell basil being added to a dish, your body may tell you "That smells perfect." When you taste curry in a dish and feel it warming your belly, you immediately know if it is good for you. When cinnamon is being baked you know if it is a good spice for you. This is certainly one area where we are wise to follow our instincts.

Fresh, organically grown spices are vastly different than the over-dried and irradiated jars of pale spices sold in many supermarkets. Freshly ground pepper is not only stronger than powdered pepper but it is also less irritating. For the fresh spices like basil, cilantro, and garlic greens, it is good to grow your own or buy them directly from the grower. For harder to grow spices like ginger or turmeric, you must shop wisely or you may get a worthless spice. Compare the smell of cinnamon between a supermarket shelf spice jar and a bin in a health food store or Indian food store and you will be amazed at the difference in potency. Generally smell and color will lead you to the best spices.

WHY SUGAR AND WHITE FLOUR ARE DAMAGING

White sugar and white flour have only appeared in the human diet relatively recently. They are not natural foods and we have not evolved to eat them. Most Americans eat a large amount of these two foods every day. White sugar and white flour contribute to many chronic diseases. Surely all of the doctor's drugs and surgeries will fail in the long run if enough of these "empty" and clogging foods are included in the diet.

White flour is what remains when the most nutritious parts of the wheat berry are removed.[57] The most nutritious part of the wheat berry is the wheat germ. The bran, which stores most of the minerals and all of the fiber, is also removed. The resulting flour is often bleached with chlorine dioxide,[58] which destroys most of the vitamin E.[59] When chlorine reacts with food, cancer-causing substances called chlorinated organics can be created.[60] There are many chemicals used to bleach and mature flour—none of them are used to promote health.

To soften white bread, ethoxylated monoglycerides and diglycerides are added. Americans eat a quarter gram a day

Some Great Cooking Spices

Ginger—warming, good for colds
Basil—cools fevers, antiviral
Thyme—kills germs and dries mucus
Black pepper—a pungent stimulant
Cinnamon—good for digestion
Sage—reduces perspiration
Garlic—prevents some infections
Cayenne pepper—a hot stimulant
Horseradish—clears sinuses
Curry—stimulates digestion
Nutmeg—numbing

of these chemicals, and no one knows exactly how harmful they might be.[61] Potassium iodate is also added to bread as a dough conditioner. Potassium iodate causes the breakdown of red blood cells and is a gastrointestinal irritant.[62] About thirty chemicals are added to help the bread look, feel, and last better. As the flour is processed, more and more chemicals are added: benzoyl peroxide, tricalcium phosphate, magnesium carbonate, calcium sulfate, and ammonium chloride. No thought is given or research done to look at the health effects of these chemicals.[63] Clearly, it is best to eat bread made from whole grains without all of these chemicals.

Both sugar and white flour contain calories of energy. Nevertheless, neither of them has the cofactors needed to burn the energy aerobically. These cofactors include coenzyme Q, coenzyme A, pantothenic acid, vitamin B2, vitamin B3, and many minerals such as zinc. If we eat a complex carbohydrate such as a whole grain we get the calories and the cofactors needed to burn the calories. However, the vast majority of these vitamins, minerals, and other cofactors are stripped out of white flour and white sugar during processing. We cannot burn the food with oxygen (aerobically), without these cofactors. So we get less energy and more fatigue. Some of the byproducts of this nonoxygen (anaerobic) energy production include lactic acid and pyruvic acid in the blood. These blood acids produce fatigue and pain.

Nutritionists and doctors are taught that one calorie is equal to another. It is wrong to think that starchy potatoes will make you fat just as quickly as chocolate cake if they have the same number of calories. When potatoes are digested, the carbohydrates are released into the blood slowly, as they are needed. When the chocolate cake is eaten, the sugar hits the bloodstream all at once. This causes the insulin reaction, which puts the extra sugar in storage. Once this glycogen storage is full, the extra sugar is converted to fat. Fat does not normally result from eating potatoes because there never is such a surplus of blood sugar.

Informed health professionals have charts of the release times and cofactor support of various carbohydrate foods to distinguish between carbohydrates. Complex carbohydrates, such as whole grains, have slower release times and the cofactors needed to make more energy. One calorie is not the same as another. The fact that complex carbohydrates release their calories slowly and the fact that cofactors are present greatly improve the value of the food.

Honey (raw, unfiltered) is different than white sugar because of the cofactors. It is also better because of traces of bee pollen, propolis, and royal jelly—especially if it is raw and unfiltered.

When we eat "empty" foods such as white flour and sugar, we get a rush of sugar into the blood. The white flour is also quickly broken down to basic sugars for rapid assimilation. But our bloodstream can handle only so much sugar. The pancreas is then forced to pour insulin into the bloodstream to put this rush of sugar into storage. And looking at a typical American on a typical white flour diet, you can see that the storage medium is fat. The sad part is that when the next energy demand is placed on this overweight person, the cofactors needed to burn the fat are missing so the fat cannot be burned. This leaves the person fat, hungry, and tired.

Obesity and pudgy fat are two of the most obvious effects of white sugar and white flour. It is destructive when overweight people use stimulants to try to speed up their metabolism to burn more fat. Without cofactors to burn the fat, it will not burn. What does burn is stored sugar and sugar in the blood until the person is even more tired. Once our systems are depleted of blood sugar, it is even harder to burn fat. Insightful health advisors will see the debilitating effects of these white foods and suggest a better diet and nutritional supplements. Many minerals are removed from white flour during processing (see the sidebar). These mineral deficiencies play a role in many diseases in America.

Another problem with white flour and white sugar is the almost complete lack of fiber. Our digestion is designed to work with fiber in our food. All natural foods have fiber. Without fiber our digestion is sluggish. One bad effect of a slow digestion is the long contact time between carcinogens

Nutrients Lost in Milling White Flour

From the USDA Nutrient Database Release 14

Compared to Whole Wheat flour,
White Wheat Flour ("enriched") has:

75% of the protein
53% of the fats
107% more calories
175% more B1 (added synthetic vitamin)
227% more B2 (added synthetic vitamin)
93% of the B3
43% of the B5
13% of the B6
59% of the folic acid
2% of the vitamin E
44% of the calcium
119% more Iron (added in a poorly absorbed form)
16% of the magnesium
18% of the manganese
31% of the phosphorus
26% of the potassium
40% of the sodium
24% of the zinc
38% of the copper
48% of the selenium
22% of the Fiber

Many other valuable constituents such as octacosanol
are removed as well.

and the bowel wall. This is a major cause of bowel cancer in those people who allow carcinogens in their food. Slowed digestion is also one cause of a host of other diseases including hemorrhoids, poor vitamin B12 uptake, lack of energy, bowel pockets and, of course, constipation.

A further problem with white flour and, to a greater extent, white sugar is blood sugar surges and dips (hypoglycemia). In a natural "complex carbohydrate" like whole grains, the sugars are released into the bloodstream slowly and regularly. Our digestion and blood sugar handling capabilities have been designed for this slow release of sugars. The short chain carbohydrates of white flour are broken down into blood sugar almost as fast as sugar.

Diabetes and hypoglycemia are in epidemic proportions in America today. Doctors know about limiting simple sugars with diabetes. Yet we need to also consider the very similar role of white flour. White bread, noodles, pastries, and a host of other items contain white flour. These same foods can be made or bought with the vastly superior complex carbohydrates of whole grains. Don't be fooled by the words "wheat flour" on a label; it means white flour.[64] "Unbleached" wheat flour is as bad as white flour except that it does not have the potentially carcinogenic residues of the bleaching process.

Each carbohydrate food has a characteristic length of time before it is released into the blood. This varies a bit between different people. In order to prevent and cure blood sugar problems, we must chart the blood sugar during the day. For instance, if a sugary breakfast is consumed, the blood sugar will rise very fast. Then the blood sugar will peak and drop. The blood sugar can be very low after one or two hours. A white flour breakfast of sugary tarts may last a couple of hours. A breakfast of whole grain complex carbohydrates can last three to four hours. Besides avoiding all of the dangers of blood sugar rushes, the complex carbohydrates will sustain you until lunchtime.

We must each chart our blood sugar swings and plan ahead to keep energetic. Planning ahead is important because when a blood sugar low is experienced, our minds do not work well. Our brains can burn only glucose for energy.[65] When our blood sugar is low, we can't think well. Health professionals can chart blood sugar based on dietary information to counsel patients on foods, mealtimes, and snacks. Smart patients are already charting their blood sugar swings.

One of the important factors leading to colds and flu is the intake of white flour. It is difficult to describe the problem to a person who has lived their whole life with a box of tissues. The white diet of Americans makes breathing through the nose a rare joy. It is true that dairy products are more powerful than white flour in thickening mucus. But the sheer bulk of white flour clogs up our mucus handling abilities. If you provide a thick mucous environment for bacteria and viruses, who can blame the germs for moving in?

Not only are whole grains much more health building than white flour, but also they each have individual qualities. Whole rye helps build muscles, whole wheat helps build energy, oats soothe irritations in the intestines, and corn builds stamina. These whole grains are called the "staff of life" because man and his ancestors have long depended on them for much of their diet.

HEALTHY FATS AND OILS

Throughout the evolution of humans, fats and oils have been difficult to find in the diet in large quantities. This is why we have an instinctive craving for them. Most fruits and vegetables have less than two percent fats, with the exception of avocados and olives, which have a higher fat content. Avocados have seventeen percent fat, and olives have eleven percent fat.[66] Whole grains range from one to seven percent fat, and nuts may contain as much as seventy percent fat.[67] Food producers and restaurants take advantage of fat cravings to get our money.

It is hard to find quality oils in a supermarket or restaurant. One of the things that makes oil undesirable is rancidity. Rancid oils taste bitter and fresh oils taste sweet. Heat, light, and oxygen in air cause rancidity. Hydroperoxides, aldehydes, and ketones are some of the irritating chemicals found in rancid oils.[68] How does oil become rancid? Frying is a great way to make oil rancid. Oils become rancid as time, heat, and oxygen convert them. Oils can also be made rancid during processing. Oil processors hide the bitter taste to cover up the rancidity. Our medical system often underestimates the role of bad oils in disease.

Quality fats and oils are needed to make hormones, to make prostaglandins, to store energy, for the nervous system, and for a host of other vital functions. With hormonal imbalances, such as premenstrual tension, the role of quality oils is important. Many women take vitamin E or evening primrose oil to aid their internal hormone production. The effects are visible as the much-needed oils are used to manufacture much-needed hormones in the body.

Of all the oils on the market, few contain both of the essential fatty acids. These essential fatty acids are called linoleic acid and linolenic acid. A healthy body can make any fat needed by using these basic building blocks. Linoleic acid is found in about one quarter of foods. The other essential fatty acid, linolenic acid, is hard to get in the diet. It is found mostly in green leafy vegetables. Evening primrose oil and the oil made from the seeds of black currants are the highest sources of linolenic acid. Flaxseed oil (*linum usitatissimum*) is the best dietary source of both essential

Nutrients Lost in Milling White Rice
From the USDA Nutrient Database Release 14

White rice has the following amounts of nutrients when compared to Brown rice:

White Rice:

25% of the fats
33% of the B3
34% of the B6
50% of the folic acid
30% of the calcium
30% of the magnesium
48% of the phosphorus
37% of the potassium
68% of the zinc
47% of the copper
34% of the manganese
17% of the fiber

A few nutrients are higher:

20% more B1
60% more B2
5% more vitamin B5
16% more energy
2.81 times more iron

Protein is the same for both

fatty acids if it is raw and properly cold processed. Oils of soybean, safflower, pumpkin, sesame, almond, avocado, and peanut have linoleic acid but just a small amount of linolenic acid.

From Soybean to Margarine

1. Pesticide residues on the plant
2. Paraquat or glyphosate used to wither the leaves just prior to harvesting
3. High temperature and pressure crushing
4. Solvents: benzene, hexane, gasoline, or carbon tetrachloride
5. Irritating additions: caustic soda, ammonia, or soda ash
6. Lecithin and vitamin E removed
7. Bleached or heated to 347 degrees Fahrenheit
8. Hydrogenation with nickel, cobalt, or copper catalyst at 400 degrees Fahrenheit. This results in trans fatty acids
9. Packed into cheap plastic bottles that leach dangerous chemicals into the oil
10. Spread on toast.

Technology has ruined many of the oils in the supermarket. Take an ordinary soybean. Because it is not an organic soybean, paraquat (a dangerous pesticide) or glyphosate (used on genetically modified soybeans) may be used to wither the leaves a week or two before mechanical harvesting. In commercial farming, the soybeans are probably already contaminated with one or more pesticides. The soybeans are crushed at high temperature and pressure and immersed in a solvent. The high temperature will produce rancidity. The solvents used in commercial production are benzene,[69] hexane, gasoline, methylene chloride,[70] and carbon tetrachloride.[71] Yes, these are poisonous or toxic and several cause cancer.[72] The solvents are removed and reused, but residues remain.

Next the soybean oil is refined with caustic soda (lye), ammonia, or soda ash. These are all irritating.[73] Lecithin is removed next to make the oil less gummy. However, lecithin is important for nerves and is a source of choline. Choline is a B-vitamin that is needed for the nerve transmitter *acetylcholine*. Next the oils are bleached or oxidized at 347 degrees Fahrenheit in a partial vacuum. All traces of vitamins A and E are removed. This is a shame, as vitamin E is needed to prevent the conversion of polyunsaturated fat into harmful peroxides in the body.[74] An antioxidant is added, such as butylated hydroxyanisole.[75] Nothing appears on the bottle of oil in the supermarket to indicate that this oil is contaminated and unnatural.

If you wanted soy margarine or shortening, hydrogenation is then done. In the presence of a catalyst of nickel, cobalt, or copper, the oil is subjected to 400 degrees Fahrenheit heat, hydrogen gas, and great pressures to make it solid. During hydrogenation some of the molecules are reversed to an unnatural form called *trans* fatty acids.[76] The chemical structure becomes a mirror image of the natural oils. This new trans chemical structure is very destructive to our cell membranes. The solid oils are then deodorized at about 500 degrees F. To top it off, the oils are packaged in cheap plastic bottles that leach chemicals into the oils.[77]

One problem with hydrogenated fats like margarine and shortening is that they contain these trans fatty acids. These trans fatty acids are not found in vegetables and are foreign to our bodies. They are, however, found in about forty percent of the foods on supermarket shelves.[78] During a recent survey of 140 varieties of crackers on a supermarket shelf, only three brands had no partially hydrogenated oil.[79]

Our cell walls regulate many important functions of transport into and out of the cell. Normal *cis* fatty acids lock together like tiny horseshoes to make this cell membrane selective. It is of critical importance for the cell membrane phospholipids to be able to regulate which chemicals will pass. The trans fatty acids are shaped like tiny lightning bolts that interfere with permeability of the cell membrane.[80] Trans fats can make cells resistant to insulin, causing obesity and diabetes.

Trans fatty acids are one cause of many diseases such as heart disease, cancer,[81] obesity, and diabetes.[82] As long ago as 1993, a Harvard Medical School study of over 80,000 nurses showed that food intake of trans fatty acids was directly related to a fifty-percent rise in the risk of coronary heart disease.[83] Trans fats were shown to increase the ratio of bad (low-density-lipoprotein) cholesterol to good (high-density-lipoprotein) cholesterol. It is the partially hydrogenated fats in vegetable shortening and margarine that are causing this rise in risk. Cookies, French fries, and white bread were also correlated with this increased risk of coronary heart disease because of their trans fatty acid content.

It is difficult, if not impossible for our bodies to burn and eliminate these unnatural trans fatty acids. I have long suspected a connection between cellulite and trans fatty acids. Nerve cells do not get their needed nutrients that have been taken out of the oils and in addition have their membranes disrupted by the unnatural oils. Margarine may be low in cholesterol, but we are wise to avoid it.

Canola oil has an interesting history. Scientists started with rapeseed oil which has toxic components. They subjected the rape seeds to intense radiation to mutate the seeds. This is a form of genetic manipulation. Some of these mutated seeds were low in toxins and high in oil content. This is how canola oil came to be made. Even organic canola oil contains these mutated genes.

The best oils are made from organic fruits or seeds and are cold pressed without solvents. These come in glass bottles or cans and should be refrigerated to reduce rancidity. When preparing something like a salad dressing, flaxseed oil or olive oil is best. For low temperature sautéing and light frying, safflower, sunflower seed, and corn oils are fine, but olive oil is healthier. For higher heat, sesame seed oil, olive oil, and peanut oil are best because they resist rancidity.

Food Addiction Syndromes

There is an interesting relationship established between people and certain foods. This relationship often involves a daily eating pattern and the cravings of addiction. It takes a long time for the cravings to diminish after the food is eliminated. The most common foods with this addictive effect in America are coffee, corn, white wheat flour, milk, sugar, and eggs.[84] Meat has similar addictions.

There is nothing inherently wrong with being addicted to foods. It may be a factor in many diseases, though. If a doctor finds that a certain food is causing a health problem or leading to a disease, the doctor is in for a challenge. People do not easily give up their addictions.

We all have a special craving for fatty foods. In a natural environment this fat craving causes no damage and is needed. After all, it is hard to crack enough nuts by hand to get a fat overload. In a modern supermarket or restaurant this fat craving leads to eating too much of the fatty and oily foods and too much of the bad kinds of fats and oils. It is these low quality fats and oils that contribute to the sixty million cases of cardiovascular disease in American people.[85]

With a natural diet of vegetables, fruits, whole grains, beans, and nuts, it is almost impossible to get too much fat or oil. The fats and oils from unprocessed natural foods also have fewer rancidity problems. Storage and burning of these natural fats and oils is easy for the body. Of course, there is no cholesterol at all in these foods. Cholesterol is only found in animal products.

Food companies take advantage of these fat cravings to sell food. The prepared food found in stores and restaurants is often very rich in fats and oils. These fats and oils are also more likely to be rancid and difficult for the body to store or burn. People enjoy the feeling of fullness that comes from eating fatty food, especially deep fried food. Stomach satisfaction is used by the food industry to sell products even though their customers are dying off.

Sugar cravings are also used by the food industry to sell products that are bad for the people who eat them. Fruit is ripe when it is sweet. That is why we have instincts to eat sweet things. Just like with fats and oils, it is hard to get too much in the way of sugars when eating a natural diet of vegetables, fruits, whole grains, beans, and nuts. It is nearly impossible to *not* get too much sugar when eating in a restaurant or when buying prepared food in a supermarket.

Most of all Americans just eat too much. It is much healthier to eat just a little *less* than enough. Destructive overeating is always bad. Of course, it is impossible to eat too much of natural, unprocessed food because we get full before we can eat too much. It is with restaurant food and empty, processed foods that overeating is a problem. Systematic under-eating is healthy if done moderately and periodically.

Chapter 7

The Ideal Environment

We must begin taking into account the toll on our health from the polluted environment of modern America. Environmental pollutants come in many forms: those we eat, those we drink, those we breathe, those our skin absorbs, chemicals at work, radiation, even noise. A complete diagnosis will include a close look at these potential causes of disease.

We exist in a country with many cancer-causing chemicals. There may be some involvement of viruses and genetic defects in cancer causation. However, those who have studied the environmental causes of cancer have found that the most prominent causes of cancer are cancer-causing chemicals and radiation.

CANCER IS CAUSED BY CARCINOGENS

The current "war on cancer" has become a misdirected waste of lives and money. The war was declared in 1971, and Americans have spent over forty billion dollars on it.[1] Cancer deaths are higher now, principally because true prevention is used so little by any part of our health care system. The five-year survival rates for all types of cancers have only improved from forty-nine to fifty-four percent since the "war" began. Another important problem is that there are more cases of cancer each year.

Cancer is rarely caused by viruses. Faulty genetics are also a rare cause of cancer. Cancer is caused by carcinogenic chemicals and also by certain types of radiation.[2] Only a small percentage of chemicals cause cancer; these should be discontinued from use. If we truly want to "kill" cancer, we must build health to resist it and avoid these carcinogens. We must also identify and remove carcinogens from our water, food, environment, and air. We must stop putting carcinogens into our environment in the first place. We must do this because once cancer has a foothold it is difficult to cure—primary prevention is the only effective course of action.

Cancer normally only occurs after a decade or more of carcinogenic abuse. There are many barriers in our bodies against the uncontrolled growth of cells. Our bodies have superb defenses against cancer. Normal cells will not reproduce unless the surrounding cells allow the growth. Tumor suppressor genes inside the cell also keep abnormal growth in check. More than half a dozen of the growth-controlling genes in a cell need to mutate in order for the cell to start toward becoming a tumor.

It is the genes in the chromosomes that can be damaged and mutate. However, chromosome damage is normally repaired by the body before cancer can occur. X-rays, other hard radiation, and certain classes of chemicals cause these mutations. Because the mutations are constantly being repaired, it often takes decades to get all of the defects to happen to one cell.

Normally, the growth-controlling genes will stop a damaged cell from reproducing. But tumors can still be triggered in several ways. Sometimes there are growth factors from outside the cell that stimulate not just one cell division, but a continuous division. Cell membranes may mistakenly stimulate cell reproduction even though they are getting no outside signals to grow. This is common in breast cancer. Some cells have internal problems that cause uncontrolled reproduction.

To stop this, the other cells surrounding a developing tumor will send braking signals to stop uncontrolled growth using tumor suppressor proteins. Our cells also have a "cell cycle clock" that stops tumor growth. This cell clock also needs to be damaged to allow tumor growth. Many redundant systems control the growth of the cell. Sometimes, though, certain viruses can disable some of these controls.

Finally, our cells will normally self-destruct if their growth regulation is damaged. Even with the constant exposure to carcinogens and the occasional exposure to hard radiation in America, tumors usually take ten to forty years to develop. Tumor development, however, is faster in children. As you can see, our defenses against cancer are very powerful.

Breast cancer is prevented by many factors such as good nutrition, avoidance of carcinogens, breast-feeding, avoiding the pill, and avoiding artificial menopausal hormones like estrogen. Mammograms do not prevent breast cancer. They detect some breast cancers in an early stage, but it is not clear if they detect them as well as or any earlier than breast self-exams, doctor exams, or breast thermography.

The powerful radiation from mammograms may also cause breast cancer. The soft tissue in breasts is especially sensitive to radiation. Breast thermography causes no harm; however, its results can be hard to interpret. Breast self-ex-

Our Defenses Against Cancer

1 Normal cells will not reproduce unless the surrounding cells allow the growth.

2 Braking signals (tumor suppressor proteins) from other cells block the growth.

3 Growth controlling genes in a cell need to mutate or no tumor can happen.

4 Tumor suppressor genes inside the cell keep abnormal growth in check.

5 Chromosomes are repaired continuously.

6 Our cells also have a "cell cycle clock" that stops tumor growth.

7 Our cells will self-destruct if their growth regulation is damaged. After 50 or 60 divisions a cell will stop reproducing.

Defects in all systems must happen in the same cell for cancer to develop.

amination is the way smart women detect problems. Instruction in breast self-exam does not prevent cancer either, but it can help to treat cancer by finding problems early. And, of course, there is no radiation damage from breast self-exams.

The use of chemotherapy drugs for cancer therapy pollutes an already contaminated cellular environment. Once breast cancer has a serious hold on a woman, modern medicine gives her only an eight percent chance of ever becoming disease free.[3] However, there are many additional ways to treat cancer that are not used in current medical practice in America. There are a large number of medicinal plants ranging from toxic *vinca rosea* (Madagascar periwinkle) and laetrile to safe red clover (*trifolium pratense*). Vitamins such as ascorbated vitamin C are of great use in cancer.[4]

Cancer is a very serious disease so careful consideration of conventional and unconventional treatments must be given. There are hundreds of natural remedies to choose from when building a complete program to cure cancer. Fasting and cleansing can be an effective part of a program if properly applied. Remember that diet plays a major role. There are excellent, health-building ways to deal with cancer instead of the dreadful drugs and burning radiation that are the standard treatment in America. If the cancer is slow growing or in an early stage there may be more time to see if these natural therapies will effect a reversal. You might consider finding an expert trained in these alternative therapies to help you decide on a course of treatment. Ideally, we will train cancer experts to understand all of the potential treatments for cancer.

ELECTROMAGNETIC RADIATION

With the universal use of computers and television, Americans are getting exposed to higher levels of electromagnetic radiation. Magnetic, electric, and microwave radiation exists in most home and work environments. This "soft" radiation contributes to a host of health problems from fatigue to cancer.[5] We can help prevent these health problems by reducing our exposure to electromagnetic radiation.

The best solution is to buy or rent a meter to detect these invisible health burdens. Medical offices could have a meter for patients to borrow. The patient can then be trained in its use and shown what levels are harmful for each type of electromagnetic radiation. The meter can be used around the home and workplace to detect high levels of electromagnetic radiation. If an electric outlet next to a child's bed is found to be high in electric radiation, the bed or outlet can be moved. If a television or computer monitor is found to be high in magnetic radiation, it can be moved away, shielded, or replaced. Children may not be safe walking under high voltage lines to school. Some fluorescent tubes emit electric and magnetic radiation. Microwave ovens and cellular phones often emit strong microwave radiation. The meter will show the correct safe distance from each of these health-depleting problems.

Microwave ovens are very common in America. They are quick and use little electricity. The standards for safety in America are one thousand times too lenient for microwave radiation leakage.[6] Most other nations have much stricter standards (one thousand times stricter) to protect the health of their people. American standards are set to protect the profits of the communications industry and to protect our defensive radar network.

Testing of microwave ovens indicates that, typically, a fifteen-foot radius around the ovens (when operating) should be maintained. This safe distance varies between different units. A bad gasket or a bit of paper in the gasket can cause severe leaks. Be careful not to use a *microwave oven test meter* unless it can measure down to 0.08 milliwatts per square centimeter because it will not be sensitive enough to find the leaks. Use a meter designed to detect microwave radiation harmful to health. Consider microwave levels over 0.08 milliwatts per square centimeter unsafe for continued exposure. The upper level of magnetic radiation for continued or repeated exposure is three milligauss. For electric exposure, three kilovolts per meter is an upper safety level. These limits are largely based upon the Swedish safety standards.

Cellular phones may be a cause of tumors.[7] The cellular phone industry has put forth studies that have looked at

---

Healthy Yards

Use fountains to cool and purify the air and sound
Have an herb garden
Use organic pest control to avoid disease
Have no mosquito breeding areas
Outside storage areas should be free from toxins
Pools and saunas should have no chlorine vapors
Child jungle gyms should not be made of treated wood
Avoid smoke from burning refuse or leaves
Use unpolluted air for exercising
Avoid exhaust and asphalt fumes

---

the effects of radio waves that are outside the cellular frequency or at exposure levels that are different from those experienced by cellular phone users. One researcher for a major cellular phone manufacturer linked cellular phones to changes in the incidence of brain tumors in rats. Newer research is showing that modern cell phones change the permeability of the blood-brain barrier, which can result in the accumulation of brain damage and lead to brain tumors.[8]

When transmitting, measurements of handheld digital cellular phones typically indicate a three-foot safe distance needed between the head and the phone. Obviously, this is too far to hear anything. Using a headset will not keep the phone's radiation away from your head. The headset acts like an antenna and transmits the microwave energy directly into the ear. This is easily checked with a testing meter. A remote mounted antenna does not reduce the amount of microwave energy emitted from the phone. Sometimes using both a wired remote antenna and a headset together can make a cellular phone safe enough for use. The antenna keeps the headset from reradiating the microwave energy into the head. Test until less than 0.08 milliwatts per square centimeter of microwave energy is received by the head. While exposure is a concern to all, it is especially important to patients recovering from tumors.

The full-spectrum light of sunlight is best for eyes and glands. All normal fluorescent tubes emit light in a very limited spectrum. If natural light is rare, our eyes can suffer. For those who must live indoors much of the time, full-spectrum bulbs or tubes are available. At least five minutes of natural light is needed daily to maintain good health. This full-spectrum light activates our hormonal system through our pineal gland.

Food Additives

To become more effective, modern medicine can look at the environment surrounding its patients. There are many factors that act upon a person's health and disease in our environment. Our bodies are able to cope with natural chemicals such as the natural defense chemicals found in plants. We are not able to cope with the thousands of unnatural chemicals in our modern environment. Over thirty-eight hundred chemicals are added to our food. Not a single one has had the rigorous testing that is required of a drug—many are not tested at all.[9]

The food industry has become a business that uses chemicals to enhance profits. These chemicals are not chosen for their healthfulness. They are chosen to make money. There are at least fifteen hundred synthetic flavorings used in food in the U.S.; France allows only six.[10] In addition to the intended additives to food, there are many unintended additives. The worst of these may be the pesticides.

To make foods pretty, food colorings are used. You may have seen the words *FD&C red #40* on ingredient labels; this coloring is used in much of the colored food in America. It has been proven to cause cancer and mutations along with Red #3, Red #4, Blue #1, Yellow #5, and Yellow #6.[11] Each time a dye is found to cause cancer, its molecule is changed a little, and we get a new carcinogen—with a new number. Many food dyes are made from aromatic amines, which come from coal tar. Some of these cause cancer directly while others break down into cancer-causing chemicals.

There are plenty of safe colorings like turmeric yellow, but they may be slightly more expensive. We must learn to protect our own health by avoiding carcinogens. Big business doesn't care about carcinogens, just profits. One chief pediatrician at Kaiser did many studies on food additives and attention deficit disorders in children. He found that the hyperactive behavior of children was often related to food additives.[12]

In some countries the list of allowable food additives is very short. In America it is vast and getting longer by the day. The average person eats fourteen pounds of food additives each year.[13] There are dictionaries of food additives.[14] If you use one, you will learn which ingredients are dangerous, which are potentially dangerous, and which are probably safe. The best way to avoid disease is to eat foods that are fresh and which have as few additives as possible. Read the labels. If you can't pronounce an additive, it is probably bad for you.

The Value of Clean Air

Fresh, clean air is very important for health. Many diseases in modern America are caused by or aggravated by bad air. Many other health problems are worsened by bad air. This bad air is found both outdoors and indoors. Throughout America there are industries, cars, and trucks emitting smog into the air we breathe. Huge clouds of smoke, soot, and pesticides move over vast areas of America.[15]

The most obvious types of health problems resulting from bad air are located in the lungs, bronchioles, nose, and sinuses. Here the air has a direct impact six million times per year. Our human respiration is able to cope with dust and dirt, and even the occasional acrid smoke. As occasional pollutants, these particles can be eliminated by healthy mucous membranes. When the pollution is continuous, as it is in cities, the pollution causes diseases. From sinus headaches to lung cancer, bad air is a major culprit.

Our mechanism for getting dirt and pollutants out of the breathing apparatus is based on the *cilia*. The cilia are tiny hair-like threads that stick up from mucous membranes in the nose, sinuses, bronchioles, and lungs. The dirt is supposed to get stuck in the mucus and then the cilia move the dirt and mucus out. Our bodies should make a thin mucus that is good for this elimination process. Dairy products, white flour, and eggs in the diet cause a thickening of this mucus.[16] The thickened mucus is less able to transport the pollutants out of the respiratory areas. Instead of continuous, effective transport, occasional colds give an explosive purging.

Our mucous membranes also suffer from dry air. Whether it is dry desert air, dry, cold, mountain air, or dry air-conditioned air, the mucous membranes are less able to eliminate air pollutants. Of course, cigarettes and other smoke also dry the mucous membranes. On the other hand, houseplants, humidifiers, baths, saunas, hot tubs, and many other solutions can be found to make the air less dry. Air conditioners and heaters can be major culprits in causing

---

Indoor Air Pollution

Pressed wood and plywood products
New rug outgassing
Pesticides
Polishes
Air conditioners and heaters
Air fresheners, cleaning fluids, or scented detergents
Second hand cigarette smoke
Fumes from fresh paint
Cooking gas fumes vented inside
House dust
Ink fumes, marking pens
Dry cleaning fumes
Perfumes
Mothproofing fumes, ammonia fumes or mothballs
Carbon paper or newspaper fumes

---

very dry air. Headaches and breathing difficulties may give way to asthma and serious lung problems over the long term.

It is important to consider these potential causes of illness when diagnosing respiratory diseases.

Indoor air pollution also causes health degradation and diseases. Tightly shut up houses, apartments, and especially mobile homes do not allow much fresh air in. The exchange rate of air in a room is the amount of time it takes for a roomful of fresh air to circulate in. With leaky old houses it can be an hour, but with modern rooms, it may take a day. The heaters or air conditioners just circulate the same old air over and over. This not only keeps pollutants in longer, but the oxygen gets depleted. Many stores have serious outgassing of toxins in their air. New houses and new furnishings often outgas formaldehyde and other toxins.[17] Air quality needs to be checked out if patients are fatigued at home. Doctors can sometimes prescribe fresh air and exercise instead of stimulant drugs.

There is a host of chemicals present in the air of a modern room. From sprayed pesticides to polishes and cleaning agents, the air may be a chemical soup. Rugs, pressboard, plywood, and clothes outgas formaldehyde, especially when new.[18] Strong chemical scents are added to many consumer products from toilet paper to detergents. Many of these chemicals can contribute to breathing problems. It is better to eliminate these causes of disease than to treat the symptoms of bad air with drugs. Doctors and their patients would be wise to become better informed about air quality.

We can do many things to improve our air. Moving to a location with a higher altitude will often help as smog tends to pool in low areas. Smell every product that you buy and let your nose decide if you should breathe the smells. Less odor is better. Never use pesticides inside a living or work area. Instead, use boric acid for cockroaches, liquid peppermint soap or cinnamon oil for ants, and other nontoxic solutions.[19] When buying new furnishings, let them air out

Environmental Exposure to Pollutants

Have you been exposed to:

_ Smoke from burning refuse or leaves.
_ Insecticide or herbicide sprays.
_ Exercise in polluted air.
_ Sprayed food.
_ Air fresheners, cleaning fluids or scented detergents.
_ Dry cleaning fumes.
_ Second hand cigarette smoke.
_ Hot dogs, food coloring, potato chips or caffeinated soda pops.
_ USDA certified colors yellow #1, blue #6, red #10, 11, 12, 13.
_ Processed meats or organ meats.
_ Food in rigid PVC containers especially oils.
_ Tap water.
_ These drugs: Flagyl, Griseofulvin, Quell, estrogen, DES, the pill.
_ Cosmetics or hair dyes.
_ X-rays or excessive, close TV.
_ Excessive sunlight.
_ Asbestos products.
_ Paint spray.
_ Workplace chemicals.
_ Fumes from fresh paint.
_ Synthetic clothing, bedding, etc.
_ Aluminum or Teflon cookware.
_ Gasoline fumes.
_ Saccharin, cyclamates and other artificial sweeteners.
_ Red meat or poultry.
_ Cooking gas fumes vented inside.
_ Housedust.
_ Air conditioning if too dry and cold.
_ Tar fumes.
_ Ink fumes, marking pens.
_ Dry cleaning fumes.
_ Perfumes.
_ Burning plastic.
_ Mothproofing fumes or mothballs.
_ Ammonia fumes.
_ Chlorine fumes.
_ Deodorants or deodorant soaps.
_ Hair dye or hair spray.
_ Automobile or diesel exhaust.
_ Carbon paper or newspaper fumes.
_ Adhesive fumes.

outside. Be careful of burning flames of propane or natural gas that vent into the breathing space. Vent them outside. Never burn treated wood.

Clean Drinking Water

Modern medicine must expand its knowledge of how contaminated water affects health and disease. Water is used to purify our bodies. It is the rain that washes us clean. The purer it is, the better it works to clean our insides. The drinking water in America does not usually contain harmful bacteria. But it often contains other harmful contaminants. There are four categories of water contaminants: germs, dirt, salts, and chemicals. Let's take a look at each type.

Germs may include parasites, bacteria, and viruses. The most common types of parasites are *Giardia lamblia, entamoeba histolytica* (traveler's dysentery), and *cryptosporidium*. They are found in some drinking water in America as well as around the world. Giardia attaches to the lining of the intestines with a pair of suckers. This attachment is made easier if the intestinal mucous lining has been stripped with copious amounts of coffee and alcohol. Neither ten minutes of boiling nor normal amounts of chlorine will kill Giardia in water. Many doctors treat Giardia with metronidazole (Flagyl®). This drug has been suspected of causing cancer and has been listed as unsafe for treatment of Giardia since before 1982.[20] The manufacturer was reported to have given the Food and Drug Administration fraudulent data to cover up the tumor-causing potential.[21] It is dangerous to use a carcinogenic drug for a self-limiting, nonfatal diarrhea. There are other natural, safer ways to treat Giardia such as with goldenseal powder (*hydrastis canadensis*).

Bacteria are largely killed off by the chlorine or bromine

treatment of American water. However, hepatitis A is a common waterborne virus in America. It is not killed by chlorine.[22] If properly engineered and maintained, ultraviolet light or ozone can kill all of these germs.

Clean Up That Water

Germs like Giardia and hepatitis A can be removed with ozone or ultraviolet light.

Dirt is removed with filters. The best filters for most uses are one to five micron spun polypropylene depth filters. Ceramic filters sized at one micron are cleanable and also remove Giardia.

Chemicals like chlorine and pesticides are best removed with granular activated carbon. The carbon works only until its adsorption sites are filled—then it is useless. You can use a pool chlorine tester on the output of a carbon filter—if it is letting chlorine through, it is exhausted.

Minerals like lead and mercury are toxic and can be removed with reverse osmosis. The best approach is to have your water tested and use a combined approach that removes the contaminants.

Dirt is often found in water and is not too harmful in itself. Dirt is composed of soil and bits of organic matter. When chlorine is added to dirty water, a group of chemicals are created which cause cancer. Some of the worst are chlorinated organic compounds such as the trihalomethanes, which are potent cancer promoters.[23]

Mineral salts are not harmful in small amounts. They are typically calcium, sodium, magnesium, and other common minerals. They are measured with an electrical resistance meter in parts per million. Seawater has about 35,000 parts per million. Drinking water usually has between one hundred and six hundred parts per million of mineral salts. Purified water has less than ten parts per million and ultra-pure water (distilled) has under one part per million.

Copper and lead are often found in solution in water that comes through distribution pipes. These are very dangerous as lead can cause mental problems in children.[24] Fluoride in the water from fluoridation can add too much fluoride to our bodies causing mottled teeth and joint disorders.[25]

Chemicals in water cause much disease, but their effects are often overlooked. The most common types of chemicals in some areas are farm pesticides. These run off into water intakes or soak into the wells. They can creep into the water supply for many years. Cancer, neurological disorders, liver damage, and a host of other problems come from pesticides in water. Much subterfuge is used by industry and government to hide the amount of pesticides in drinking water. For example, California keeps a pesticide database for wells. All of the single positive tests for pesticides by certified labs are thrown out if a later test does not confirm the amount.[26] Because the pesticide amounts vary from time to time, thousands of positive readings are thus hidden from the public. In addition to farm pesticides, industrial sources often introduce dangerous chemicals into the public water supply.

Doctors can find out if their communities' water supply is contaminated. They also can find out which methods are best for removing the contamination. Filtration takes out dirt, but is of little help with chemicals, salts, or bacteria.

Reverse osmosis takes about ninety-six percent of everything out except harmful chemicals. Activated carbon removes chlorine, trihalomethanes, and pesticides until the cartridge is depleted. Once the adsorption sites in the carbon are filled, no further chemicals are removed. Ultraviolet light or ozone gas can be used to sterilize water. Bottled water quality varies from excellent to just tap water. If the bottle says, "purified," then it is likely to be drinkable. "Spring water" or "drinking water" bottles may just be ordinary tap water, or they may be purified.

We don't just drink the tap water, either. When cooking, some of the chemicals are in the steam. When showering with hot water, we breathe the chemicals; the chlorine or bromine smell can be overpowering. Hot tubs and swimming pools can have a layer of harmful gas right where you are breathing. The effect on skin of the chemicals and the acidity of the water should also be considered. The best dermatologists know about the effects of water pollutants on the skin.

PART III

HOW TO MAKE MEDICAL CARE SAFER

Chapter 8

Perilous Prescriptions

Thousands of tons of pills are consumed every year by Americans.[1] Approximately 3.5 billion prescriptions were filled in the United States in 2002![2] Our whole medical system is based upon drugs. It would be safer if medical schools were to emphasize changing lifestyle habits and prescribe healthy diets for patients. Common medical approaches are to attack a problem in the body with drugs or with surgery. Drugs are also used to regulate chemical reactions inside of our bodies.

Drugs can work miracles and save many lives when used judiciously. When drugs are used for minor diseases, however, the side effects can sometimes be worse than the original disease. We must learn how to build a strong, disease-free health and use drugs only when safer methods have failed or when there is an emergency.

The United States General Accounting Office found that more than half of the drugs approved by the FDA were later found to have severe or fatal side effects. These side effects were not found during the FDA's review and testing. More than half of all drugs approved during the nine-year period studied had to be taken off of the market or required major label changes due to missed safety issues.[3] Doctors can continue to prescribe these drugs long after they are found to be dangerous.

There is a strong analogy between a drug approach to killing germs in the body and a pesticide approach to killing bugs in the field. Both a vigorously healthy body and a vigorously healthy field of plants can resist disease. Drugs and pesticides do not promote this strong health and resistance. Instead they undermine the health of the person and the health of the soil. With chemical agriculture the soil becomes worse and so more pesticides are needed. The same is true of drugs and people. While a drug treatment may be helping a specific health problem, it can also be decreasing the overall health of the person. Furthermore, the bacteria in the body become resistant with antibiotic therapy just like the pests in the field become resistant to pesticides. Chemical companies don't prevent pests; they just sell chemicals to get rid of the pests. Drug companies don't prevent disease; they just sell drugs to get rid of the disease. Primary prevention is not part of these businesses and prevention is not good for their success.

There are just too many drugs on the market. Experienced clinicians know that vastly fewer drugs would be enough for ninety-nine percent of health problems.[4] Health Maintenance Organizations (HMOs) are recognizing this with their formularies. A formulary is a restricted list of drugs that the HMO doctors can prescribe without special per-

mission. Truly new drug discoveries have been on the decline since the 1950s. Variants of the old drugs come out in
new combinations constantly, which results in more drugs.
It would be safer to have fewer drugs so that more testing
for long-term effects could be done. Genetic engineering may
be coming up with new drugs, but we have yet to see what
the side effects of this type of drug will be.

Pesticides	Drugs
Kill pests in the field	Kill pests in the body
No need with strong plants	No need with strong health
Lowers health of the field	Lowers health of the body
Worse soil needs more sprays	Worse health needs more drugs
Creates resistant bugs	Creates resistant germs

Organic growing builds better soil. It costs more in the
short term and saves money in the long term. Natural
health also takes more effort at first and saves much pain
and cost later.

Drugs save many lives and are effective in controlling
many health problems. Yet, we should be cautious in using
them as almost 100,000 deaths and two million injuries each
year are attributed to adverse reactions to drugs prescribed
by doctors.[5] These numbers of adverse reactions excluded

errors due to drug administration, noncompliance, overdose, drug abuse, and therapeutic failures.

From five to nine percent of the patients in American hospitals are there as a direct result of adverse reactions to prescription drugs.[6] Even more people are admitted to hospitals because of various medication problems.[7] Over three billion dollars are lost every year because of medication problems. Much of this is preventable.

That unintelligible scrawl that is the emblem of many doctors creates some of this treatment-caused disease. Many drugs have similar names. An illegible prescription can result in the wrong drug being used. Half of the handwritten and oral orders of doctors were found to be unclear. This is a major cause of drug overdose.[8] Fewer than one quarter of doctors' orders for intravenous fluids were found to have enough instructions to administer the fluid properly.[9] Doctors sometimes do not look up the correct dosage. For instance, tetanus shots were prescribed at the wrong dosage one quarter of the time in an emergency room study.[10] Nurses and doctors can also make calculations that result in wrong dosages.[11] These communication breakdowns can ruin lives. To a certain extent, some of the newer digital handheld technologies can be helpful in clearly spelling out orders and performing calculations, thereby eliminating these problems. The real problem is that our medical system uses too many dangerous drugs too often.

One of the problems with the chemical drug approach is that the body resists the drugs. There is a two-phased response to most drugs. At first the drug will do the job, it seems. After a while, the body will adapt to the drug or try to block it. This adaptation or blocking creates a vicious cycle where the drug can worsen the problem it was intended to cure. If we take insulin, our body will make less insulin to compensate; we become dependent. Over time we need more and more. If we take anabolic steroids, our body will make less of the male hormones; the big muscles look good at first, but later there may be reduced hormone output.[12] If we take SSRI (Selective Serotonin Reuptake Inhibitor) drugs, such as some mood-enhancers like Prozac, our own ability to make serotonin from tryptophan may be weakened.

Short-term or emergency medicine saves many lives with drugs. However, for the chronic health problems that make up the vast majority of medical situations, these drugs can do more harm than some safer natural therapies. Drugs are not intended to build long-term vibrant health. It is difficult for a purely drug approach to achieve true healing of chronic or degenerative diseases.

TREATMENT-CAUSED ILLNESS IS

UNNECESSARY

Well-intentioned doctors are causing pain, disability, and death in epidemic numbers using today's medical approaches. While our current medical system saves many lives and helps millions of people, this system also causes much agony. Most treatment-caused deaths and injuries are the result of drug reactions and drug side effects. Medical devices and hospital infections cause many more of these injuries.

Much of the current drug use is unnecessary. Whereas the drugs of modern medicine do sometimes cause bad side effects, natural therapies normally do not. The number of deaths from treatment-caused disease is greater than that from traffic accidents and industrial accidents.[13] We must become smart enough to use less harmful therapies whenever possible.

Treatment-caused disease is a major problem in our hospitals. There are more hospital beds devoted to hospital-acquired infections than are devoted to either accidents or cancer.[14] These infections are among the top ten leading causes of death in the US. These infections cost over 2.5 billion dollars each year.[15] Many of the hospital-acquired infections are preventable.

The medical term for treatment-caused illness is *iatrogenic* illness. There are several types of treatment-caused illnesses. One kind is when a doctor makes a mistake. The doctor may give the wrong drug or the wrong dose. Another kind of treatment-caused illness is when the doctor gives the correct dose of a medically correct drug, but there are side effects. These are the risks of modern medicine. However, these are not the risks of many other healing modalities. These are often unnecessary risks.

More and more prescriptions are being given out.[16] Between 1985 and 1999, using data from the National Ambulatory Medical Care Survey, the prescription rate increased from 109 to 146 prescriptions per 100 visits.[17] An average hospitalized person gets thirteen different drugs.[18] This use of many drugs at once is called *polypharmacy* or "shotgun prescription." Some of these drugs may be prescribed by different doctors who are unaware of the other drugs.[19] This makes bad drug interactions all too common. Modern artificial intelligence is beginning to be used to screen drugs to forestall many of these interactions.

Many times people come to doctors with problems that drugs cannot help. In some cases a prescription is written anyway.[20] This may be done to satisfy patient expectations or as a kind of ritual—instead of for the good of the patient. The trend now is for the common drugs to be stocked right in the doctor's office. This may increase a doctor's income.[21] However, it may be safer to have a pharmacist overseeing the prescriptions.

Forty percent of people getting medical care develop adverse side effects from their medications.[22] One reason that this happens is that toxic levels of drugs vary widely between different people.[23] The number and variety of miseries caused by side effects of drugs is vast. People tend to accept these side effects as inevitable. They are usually not inevitable. There are often a number of alternatives to drug therapy.

Treatment-caused illness is a common reason for hospitalization—especially for the elderly, children, or infants. Twenty-eight percent of hospital admissions are due to various prescription drug-related problems including adverse reactions.[24] The number of treatment-caused deaths each year from direct and indirect effects is reported to be as high as 250,000 people.[25] Many of these deaths are unnecessary. Many more patients don't die, but are maimed and poisoned by the drugs of modern medicine.

Drug Side Effects

All drugs damage or stress your body in some way. This is because they are not natural. Our bodies have not evolved to deal with these artificial substances. Because the drugs are synthesized and concentrated, our senses of smell and taste do not protect us from their effects. Many drugs are designed to act quickly. This rapidity of action makes them more dangerous. If you take too much of a medicinal plant remedy you are likely to be warned by your senses or by feeling nauseous. Our bodies have evolved with these plant remedies and can usually warn us if we need to lower the dose. Overdosing with pharmaceuticals is all too easy.

If you must take a drug, get acquainted with the side effects by reading the Physician's Desktop Reference book (PDR). See if your pharmacist can give you a complete list of the drug's side effects by photocopying the PDR. Other sources of side-effect information such as the Internet are often simplified to hide drug dangers. Pharmacy computer printouts also can be a shortened list of the side effects.

Note carefully the side effects that signal danger. Check carefully to see if carcinogenic (cancer-causing) effects have been tested. Better yet, find a doctor who can suggest natural alternative remedies and recommend healthful changes in your habit patterns.

High blood pressure drugs are good examples of drugs with terrible side effects. Many of these antihypertensive drugs cause impotence in men and sexual dysfunction in women.[26] They cause a long list of unpleasant side effects. Drug-oriented medicine can prescribe these drugs even for borderline cases of high blood pressure. The patient may not even have had high blood pressure before going into the doctor's office. Nervousness when entering a doctor's office or clinic can easily raise blood pressure.

When a person has high blood pressure, it is really his or her lifestyle that is causing the problem. Changing towards a more vegetarian diet with less salt is very effective. Relaxation techniques and stress control help tremendously. Less work and more exercise are prescriptions that work and have beneficial side effects. Patients need an explanation as to the dangers of the drugs and the benefits of the lifestyle changes. When faced with a clear choice, patients can make a conscious decision. They can choose to make the lifestyle changes needed and become happier and more fit. Or, they can choose to use the drugs for life with the risk of impotence and other side effects.

Today, millions of people are taking multiple drugs. The side effects from the various drugs add to or multiply the side effects of other drugs. One way this happens is when one drug lessens the ability of the liver to detoxify the other drugs. Our liver is needed for neutralizing some drug toxins. We can often find ways to treat health problems with fewer drugs. If multiple drugs really must be used, patients should research the interactions of their drugs.

Drug-oriented medicine is at the root of an epidemic of sedatives, mood elevators, and tranquilizers. Prozac, Zoloft, and Paxil are some of the most overprescribed drugs. Over sixty million Valium prescriptions are written each year. It is interesting that Valium's side effects (confusion, mood changes, depression, tremors, and restlessness) are often the same as some of the reasons for taking it.[27] Valium and barbiturates are responsible for a large percentage of drug abuse deaths.

RESPONSIBLE PRESCRIBING

Drug companies spend an average of $26,000 each year on each doctor to convince them to prescribe their drugs.[28] The information given to doctors about the drugs is filtered by the drug company detail men that see the doctors.[29] The drug companies do the drug testing. The drug companies pay for the clinical test reports. The drug companies pay for the research grants that result in medical journal papers. This system is not working toward safer drugs. Thirty-five percent of complaints against clinical trials checked by the FDA (United States Food and Drug Administration) were for protocol violations. Another twenty-four percent were for falsification of data.[30] A recent study of clinical trials of drugs concluded that these drug tests are frequently incomplete and biased. Harmful drug reactions were incompletely reported in 65% of the cases studied.[31]

It is doctors who have the responsibility to prescribe drugs responsibly. The drug companies put all of the side effects in the Physician's Desktop Reference (PDR) to protect themselves from litigation. Busy doctors can reduce drug problems by checking the package inserts or the PDR for side effects.

One classic example of overprescribing a dangerous drug is chloramphenicol.[32] During the 1960's this drug brought in about one third of a major pharmaceutical company's overall profits. It was already reported that people who took this drug stood a chance of dying from aplastic anemia. Only for certain cases of typhoid is this powerful and dangerous drug really needed. This drug company spent large sums to promote their profit-making drug. Doctors were persuaded to prescribe it four million times a year for minor problems such as acne, colds, sore throat, and infected hangnails. Hundreds of people died.[33]

After a Congressional hearing, the drug company was forced to put strong warnings in with the drug. Exports of the drug were exempt from warning labels so the profits of the drug company continue to roll on in foreign countries.[34] Responsible doctors do their own research and refuse to prescribe terrible drugs like this one. These doctors make medicine safer by eliminating this cause of unnecessary deaths and injuries.

It takes only a few minutes to write a prescription. It takes longer to counsel the patient as to lifestyle, fitness, diet, and individual problems. Drugs are often given to hide a problem, most commonly pain. Pain is the body's way of telling us that something is wrong. Ignoring and suppressing any of these warning signals is dangerous. While suppressing pain is sometimes necessary, we must also look at healing the cause of the pain.

When people are drugged all of the time, it takes away some of their aliveness and can stifle their consciousness. The pharmaceutical corporation's toolbox is creating an anesthetized society. This widespread anesthesia creates a de-mand for ever-greater stimulation from noise, speed, and violence.

Doctors may sometimes prescribe a drug to satisfy pa-tient expectations. However, studies show that many patients want more herbal remedies, massage, and discussion of safe and natural alternatives.[35] The best doctors are moving more in that direction.

DRUG SAFETY

There are many reasons why some drugs turn out to be dangerous after testing and licensing. After a period of time, our body resists the effects of many drugs. This may be be-cause our body learns to produce more of the chemical that the drug is blocking. It may be that our body learns to make less of the chemical that the drug is replacing. Our body may resist the drug by changing the effectiveness of the en-zymes affected. Our body may alter transport of the drug across cell membranes. Clinical tests often miss these sec-ondary effects because the tests are of too short a duration to catch them.[36]

Another obvious reason that some drugs are declared dangerous after use is that they are poorly tested. The drug company that will make millions on the drug is the same company that tests the drug. Careers often depend upon a researcher verifying his or her own discovery. Clinical tests are rife with corruption.[37] Much important information has been suppressed. Even the well-tested drugs are subject to the body's adaptation.

We all remember Thalidomide, the pregnancy sedative that caused so many terribly malformed babies. Another drug, reserpine, is still used for high blood pressure despite the fact that it has been reported to double the risk of breast cancer.[38] Drug disasters with drugs such as Vioxx are going

Problems with Antibiotics

Bacteria become resistant
Impairment of the immune system
Will kill some healthy bacteria in intestines and else-where
Overuse, preventive use, and casual use
Used on viruses where they do no good
Can cause yeast infections
Terrible side effects from stronger antibiotics
Allergic reactions
Don't build the immune system
Lead to antibiotic dependency

They do not address susceptibility and
the causes of infection

on all the time. Diethylstilbesterol (DES) was used to treat menstrual disorders until it was found to cause vaginal cancer.

In comparison, most medicinal plants have been available for hundreds or thousands of years. Only a handful of the hundreds of medicinal plants have been found to pose dangers.

ANTIBIOTICS

At one time "miracle" antibiotics saved lives. They still save lives, but now these wonder drugs can also threaten health. One of the real dangers is *superinfection*. This occurs when bacteria become resistant to an antibiotic. More and stronger antibiotics are needed to fight these resistant bacteria. For the same infection, up to fifty times as much penicillin is needed today than was needed thirty years ago.[39] Some bacteria are evolving to become resistant to all antibiotics. The most resistant types of bacteria live in hospitals. Some antibiotics impair the immune system, leaving the person more vulnerable to infection after the antibiotics.[40] The overuse of antibiotics leaves the bacteria stronger and the patients with weakened immune systems.

The Centers for Disease Control and Prevention estimate that there are fifty million unnecessary antibiotic prescriptions written each year.[41] Prescriptions for antibiotics are given 150 million times per year in America.[42] This overprescribing of antibiotics is often done over the phone or without any tests.[43] This overprescribing of antibiotics may be the most important cause of candida vaginitis and other yeast infections.[44] The use of powerful broad-spectrum antibiotics is even more dangerous because a wider spectrum of bacteria is encouraged to become resistant. Because many lifesaving surgical procedures depend on antibiotics, this overuse of antibiotics will make these procedures more and more dangerous. Sometimes antibiotics are prescribed as a preventive measure. Using antibiotics for prevention is of debatable value and can make the patient more vulnerable to later infection. There are often other, safer solutions that stop infections.

There are a limited number of antibiotics possible. Truly

new antibiotics are becoming rare. The modifications of ex-
isting antibiotics are losing their effectiveness. Stronger antibiotics are being used because germ resistance is building
to the common antibiotics. No truly new anti-staphylococ-
cus antibiotics have been developed for a quarter of a century. Vancomycin is perhaps the last antibiotic left to which
certain staphylococcus infections respond. Note that it costs
$800 a day and can cause terrible side effects such as deaf-
ness.[45] Even with Vancomycin, resistance to the antibiotic
increased 700 times in certain bacteria over a four-year period.[46]

The vast use of antibiotics in animal feed is also contributing heavily to the problem of bacterial resistance. Those
who touch raw meat can cause their bacteria to become resistant to antibiotics. Most residents of the United States
eat low levels of antibiotics in meat, eggs, and dairy products throughout their entire lifetimes.[47] The antibiotics found
in these foods are the same antibiotics that are used as medicine. Special antibiotic markers used in the creation of genetically modified food also can cause resistant bacteria.

However, there are many natural antibiotics from medicinal plants such as Goldenseal, Usnea, and Garlic. We
can use these medicinal plant solutions coupled with plants
like Echinacea and Larch that stimulate the immune system
to fight staphylococcus and other infections. These medicinal plants do not cause bacterial resistance to build up. Instead, they work with the body to fight infection.

Dietary change and colon cleansing are also important
in fighting infection. Ascorbated vitamin C is a powerful tool
in fighting infections. There are medicinal plants that lower
fever. There is a wealth of information about fighting infections using natural means from all of history and all around
the world. This information is not used to its full potential
by our current medical system.

Despite the fact that penicillin and other antibiotics are useless against viral infections like colds and flu, they are often prescribed for these conditions. Every year about eighteen million Americans get an antibiotic prescription for a cold.[48] Without gaining any benefit in relieving the cold, these patients are left open to side effects and superinfections.

Allergic reactions to penicillin range from bothersome rashes to deadly anaphylactic shock.[49] Spectinomycin costs six times as much as penicillin and may have even more side effects. Chloromycetin is a powerful antibiotic developed for meningitis and typhoid. It interferes with the bone marrow's production of blood.[50] It is harmful to prescribe this for children's sore throats. It does not help with a viral sore throat and can create a need for multiple transfusions. Tetracycline is often prescribed for colds. Residues may accumulate in the bones and teeth, especially in children under eight years of age.[51] It is of extremely dubious effectiveness for the cold itself.

Most importantly, reliance on antibiotics misses addressing the cause of the susceptibility to infection. Look for doctors who will help you to become stronger, thereby stopping the cycles of infections and antibiotics.

STEROID HORMONES

Steroid drugs are another of the powerful wonder drugs that have become overused. They mimic the action of the adrenal hormones or other hormones to powerfully affect body systems. They are now prescribed for common conditions such as acne, inflammations, and sunburn. They are even used for bodybuilding. It is better to find ways to support the natural production of the body's own hormones instead of using steroid drugs. For instance, vast research indicates that *panax ginseng*, a root from China, safely stimulates endocrine hormone production.[52]

The side effects of one commonly used steroid drug, prednisone, are very harmful. There are dozens of bad side effects from prednisone. This drug should be used only as a last resort. Why give this drug for a skin inflammation while there are so many safe alternatives? For example, aloe vera gel (*aloe Barbadensis*), green clay, and calendula tea (*calendula officinalis*) are all used externally to soothe skin inflammations without harmful side effects.

The "pill" is another steroid hormone prescribed for over ten million American women—about one billion worldwide. It fools the body into thinking it is pregnant. The risk of cardiovascular disease by women over forty taking the pill is much higher than it is for women who do not take the pill. All women on the pill are at increased risk for liver tumors, headaches, depression, and cancer.[53] The risk of high blood pressure is six times greater, the risk of stroke four times greater, and the risk of blood clots five times greater because of clotting problems.[54] There are safe, natural alternatives. Men can be trained to control pregnancy without drugs.

Women are also a target for menopausal *hormone replacement therapy*. Estrogen (sometimes with progestin) is prescribed for over five million women in America. It has been recently found that hormone replacement therapy increases the risk of breast cancer, heart attacks, strokes, and blood clots.[55] Long-term use of hormone replacement therapy also increases a woman's chance of ovarian cancer by three hundred percent.[56] It has been found to do more harm than good.[57] Yet today's doctors have been prescribing this dangerous drug for the most minor of menopausal discomforts. Some doctors even insist that their women patients over age thirty-five take hormone replacement therapy, no matter what symptoms may or may not be present. This practice is changing, however, as evidence mounts on the dangers of hormone replacement therapy.

It makes more sense to prescribe evening primrose oil and exercise for hot flashes. There are also excellent medicinal plant formulas to alleviate the symptoms without bad

Solutions for Hyperactive Kids and Attention Deficit Disorder

More exercise and outdoor fun
Quality snacks and good food
More interesting classes
Less computer and TV time
Reduced food additives and coloring
Reduced sugar and no caffeine
Gardening and pets
Warm family support

side effects. One of the most effective herbal formulas for hot flashes contains black cohosh (*cimicifuga racemosa*), blessed thistle herb (*cnicus benedictus*), false unicorn root (*helonias dioica*), panax ginseng, licorice root, sarsaparilla (*smilax officinalis*), and squaw vine (*mitchella repens*). Results are usually rapid, and there are no bad side effects.

It is ironic that our medical system still recommends estrogen for the prevention of depression and cardiovascular disease even though estrogen has been proven to be ineffective for these conditions. Estrogen is also still used to prevent osteoporosis. It is smarter to use diet and exercise to prevent osteoporosis, rather than increasing cancer risk.

Psychiatric Drugs

It is all too easy for a child to become drug dependent. Many drugs come not from a schoolyard drug dealer, but from the pharmacist. If a kid is a little too energetic for a teacher's taste, the child is in danger of becoming medicated. Millions of children are the unwilling recipients of psychiatric drugs.[58] The usual reason given for using these drugs is that the child is hyperactive or has attention deficit disorder. Even a flimsy diagnosis may result in a drugged child. Many schools receive thousands of dollars for each child taking drugs for attention deficit disorder. With public school funds diminishing constantly, what school could just say no to this offer?

If a child doesn't pay attention in class, medicine's first solution is drugs. A more interesting curriculum might better solve the problem. Hunger and fatigue cause much of the inattention in class. The usually prescribed drugs have bad side effects such as suppression of growth, high blood pressure, nervousness, and insomnia. Drug companies are influencing doctors to prescribe these drugs for children. These companies are making millions from over-drugged children.

Parents of overactive children should know about Dr. Feingold's research into the causes of hyperactivity in children. As chief of the allergy clinics for Kaiser, he noted that food coloring and food additives often contribute to child hyperactivity. Exercise and fun are obvious cures for peppy children. Parents should consider that five hours sitting in class and another eight hours behind a TV or computer have something to do with hyperactivity. Perhaps a diet loaded with sugar and caffeine contributes. Maybe a lack of warm family support and too much isolation contributes to hyperactivity. We must find solutions that help and don't hurt.

It is not only children that receive too many prescriptions for psychiatric drugs. The drug approach to psychological imbalance should not be the first way to treat mental illness in adults, either. There are real reasons for mental imbalance. We must take a closer look at the reasons for the imbalance and recommend real solutions that change the causes of these problems. Many of the comments mentioned above on child problems also apply to adults. Good nutrition with a custom-designed supplement schedule can help many mental/emotional problems. Stress relief programs are effective, especially coupled with a good fitness program. Drugs should be the last resort, not the first thing tried.

Personal Care

In the past, doctors treated people who they knew personally. They considered each person as an individual. Ethics and morals guided them to cause as little harm as possible. Now some doctors behave more like scientific technicians treating classes of diseases instead of individuals. Treatment-caused illness is now seen as just an error in the medical machine. It is best if your doctor knows and cares for you personally. Having a personal physician is difficult in this age of managed health care.

Malpractice is legally defined as a doctor not acting according to the medical code. It is not considered malpractice to ignore excellent natural treatments used throughout the world. It is not malpractice to prescribe drugs that cause great harm if it is normal medical practice to do so. It is not considered malpractice to subject people to unnecessary operations. Most of treatment-caused illness is not technically malpractice. It is time that we examine even medically accepted treatments for potential dangers.

Attempts to avoid malpractice suits are now a leading cause of treatment-caused illness. Diagnostic tests can be given to ward off a possible malpractice suit even when the tests are invasive, damaging, and unnecessary.

We have all been raised to know that drug therapy can have very positive effects. We also need to realize that drugs can have temporary effects and severe side effects. The best solutions to health problems often involve changing our health choices. Drugs should only be used as a backup to safer natural therapies.

Chapter 9

Healing Hospitals

Imagine arched walkways filled with fragrant and beautiful flowers. Imagine a deep silence and peace interrupted only by the occasional call of a bird or cricket. A friendly massage therapist comes to relax your muscles for sleep. Imagine a place where balance is restored and the body is cleansed. You are consoled, cared for, and comforted in a secure, relaxed environment.

Imagine a place where you are treated with respect and dignity. Imagine consulting as equals with men and women of knowledge and wisdom. Here you can learn all about your health problem, how it came to be, and how it will be resolved. Mobilize your self-healing powers. Learn the wonders of the self-repairing body and how Mother Nature heals.

When you are strong enough, gardens wait to inspire and strengthen you. From the gentlest exercise you are gradually moved toward strength. Strange but tasty food leaves you with a warm, satisfied feeling. Imagine deep, fragrant baths, sometimes hot and sometimes cool and refreshing. Become reunited with the rhythms of nature.

Hospital Dangers

Our hospitals have become something quite different from this idyllic vision. Peace and dignity are hard for patients to maintain in a hospital. Patients seem transformed into limp and mystified spectators of their own treatment. Loudspeakers and machines constantly interrupt healing rest. How can one call upon the healing power of nature when one is so far removed from nature? Our medical system may work hard to help us, but only nature can perform the miracle of healing.

We must work to make hospitals safer places. It is important to stop the breeding of antibiotic-resistant bacteria. Heating and cooling ducts can spread infection to weakened patients. Sheets are changed between patients now, but the pillows and mattress pads also need to be changed to prevent infection. Staff members of the hospitals need to be careful so that they are not collectors and distributors of microorganisms. Contaminated devices are responsible for many hospital infections.

If hospitals used effective disinfectants and sanitary protocols, then three-quarters of the 100,000 deaths from infection each year could be prevented.[1] Two million patients each year acquire an infection while in a hospital in America.[2] Hospital death rates have doubled in the last fifteen years. One study showed that forty-two percent of hospital deaths were preventable for those admitted with a low severity of illness.[3] Except for surgery, doctors have been found to wash

Hospital Checklist

- Bring a pillow, bathrobe, and slippers
- Bring vitamins and supplements
- Bring healthy foods and superfoods
- Bring books, notepaper, and pens
- Bring nonstressful reading material
- Bring headphones and favorite music
- Bring earplugs and an eye mask
- Bring a friend
- Check if your procedure can be
  done as an outpatient
- Check each pill and dose
- Check each IV
- Check medications for interactions
- Check medications for dangerous side effects
- Check for harmful diagnostic procedures
- Check each device for contamination
- Check for unnecessary x-rays
- See if less radical surgery is possible
- Make sure your doctors and nurses wash their hands
  or change gloves before touching you
- Check how long your doctor has been on call
- Ask the nurses which is the best doctor for you
- Check the infection rate for the hospital
- Check the mortality rate for your procedure
- Check the rate of medication error
- Check to see that you are not in a clinical trial
- Visualize a positive outcome

their hands only half the time between patients in hospitals.[4] Because hospitals are now a business, the housecleaning staffs are kept to a minimum. Many of these problems occur because stockholders' profits are seen as more important than patient care.

There are many ways to make our hospitals safer. Patients receive an average of over a dozen different prescription drugs.[5] Patients should have fewer drugs and have better communication with prescribing doctors. Care is required to prevent mix-ups such as the wrong operation or the wrong medications. There is so much electronic equipment that electric shocks are a possibility. Electronic interference with monitoring equipment may happen as well. Proper storage of chemicals, solvents, and radioactive wastes is essential to prevent the possibility of contamination. Invasive and damaging diagnostic procedures should be avoided when possible. These diagnostic procedures account for some of our treatment-caused illness.[6]

Malnutrition has been found in twenty-five to fifty percent of patients in studies of American and British hospitals.[7] Average hospital diets supply too little of many important minerals and vitamins including the vital antioxidant vitamins. This malnutrition combined with the other stressors in the hospital is a recipe for health disaster. Our immune systems depend on vitamins and minerals to function. Hospital patients are malnourished because the food contains too few nutrients and also because patients tend to eat too little.[8] More fresh food and supplements can help.

DIGNITY IN THE HOSPITAL

There is an unnecessary assault on human dignity in hospitals. The assembly line approach to dealing with sick people can be insensitive. Patients' clothes are taken away and they are given a flimsy nightshirt that is open in the back. It would help to allow the patient to bring a freshly laundered bathrobe. Patients should be allowed to sit up in chairs if it will not hurt their therapy. Patients should be allowed to walk if they are capable of walking instead of being wheeled around on gurneys or in wheelchairs. These procedures inevitably humiliate and demean people. It is best when hospital staff at least appear to consult with their patients. No one likes to be ordered around.

Hospital staff members must not become hardened to the trials of their charges. Patients should never be reduced to a number and a symptom. We should avoid an atmosphere of fear and despair. It is common for patients to feel abandoned because they are separated from their family. Fear suppresses their immune system. We need hospitals, but they need to be better, safer, and more pleasant hospitals.

HOSPITAL BIRTH

Hospital-born babies are more likely to suffer distress during labor and delivery, get caught in the birth canal, need resuscitation, get infected, or have hemorrhaging mothers than those borne at supervised home births.[9] This may be partly because the most difficult births happen in hospitals. Home births attended by a trained midwife or doctor are just as safe as hospital births.[10] More than ninety percent of births have no complications in supervised home births.[11] The shaving, the episiotomy, the IV (intravenous fluids), the forced position in the stirrups, the strangers watching, the lack of family present, and the sterile atmosphere add up to an unpleasant experience. With a supervised home birth, many of these procedures are found to be unnecessary. Midwives often have lubricating and relaxing oils that are used instead of an episiotomy. Women have more choices in position with a home birth. Birthing rooms in hospitals are a solution to many of these concerns. Family can be present and infection is less of a concern in a birthing room.

The American College of Obstetricians and Gynecologists has taken a stand against home birth. They quote statistics that give the impression that there are four times as many stillbirths outside of hospitals. This is only true if you include accidental and unattended births.[12] Consider that only six percent of midwives have been sued for malpractice.[13] This statistic is very steady over the years.[14] However, seventy percent of obstetricians have been named in malpractice suits.[15] The best situation is when a trained midwife can attend a home birth with a doctor present or on call for problems. If complications are expected, a hospital birth makes more sense than a home birth.

Having the baby taken away from the mother right after birth is a travesty against nature. Formula feeding is also highly detrimental to the child and mother. These bad practices are perpetuated without good reason. Supportive doctors help their patients have their baby at home and encourage breast-feeding whenever possible.

Modern medicine needs to become more aware of the benefits of breast-feeding. Breast milk contains antibodies to infectious diseases that the mother has come in contact with. Breast milk has a changing spectrum of nutrients that perfectly match the infant's needs. Important bonds are formed between mother and child with breast-feeding. The mother benefits from a lowered risk of breast cancer, and she makes more hormones to shrink the uterus just after birth. Formula-fed infants are plagued by a host of diseases including ear infections, diarrhea, and respiratory infections.[16] Infant formula and commercial baby food lack vital enzymes and nutrients and often contain too much sugar and salt and too many additives. It is a very bad practice to give a free six-pack of formula to each new mother.

Hospital Death

We can improve the experience of hospital death by allowing the presence of the family. Personal dignity is easier to find in a home death. Peacefulness is also easier to find at home. While modern medicine itself struggles with death, the patient can be left as a helpless observer. At home a person can preside at his or her own death and decide when to go. It is better to die surrounded by loved ones than to die in impersonal surroundings and loneliness.[17] When death becomes inevitable, the patient should be able to choose when, where, and how to die. Better hospitals recognize this and send the patient to a hospice or home for their last farewells.

Hospital Survival Tips

If you must go to a hospital, take a friend or relative to protect you from the psychological and physical dangers. Your partner can make sure you are nourished and comforted. Your partner can make sure that you get the right pills, surgery, x-rays, and IV drip.

Try to minimize the number and potency of your medications in the hospital. Also limit the tests to just the ones that you really need. It is wise to build your immune system up before entering a hospital. Make sure your doctors and nurses change their gloves or wash their hands before touching you. One of the most important questions to ask your doctor in the hospital is how many hours he or she has been on call. If the doctor has been on call for more than ten or twenty hours, request a fresh doctor. You may want to ask the nurses to direct you to the best doctor. They often know which doctor will give you the best service.

If possible find out the infection rate for the hospital; it really does vary. Find out the mortality rate for the procedure proposed. Find out the rate of medication error. You might consider getting a written response indicating that you are not involved in any research or a clinical trial. This information is often hard to obtain.[18]

BACK TO THE HOUSES OF HEALING

What can be done about the state of our hospitals? The obvious goal is to keep as many people as possible out of hospitals. Home care removes most hospital problems and can surround the patient with loved ones. Outpatient care is a solution for many problems and most convalescence.

Hospitals used to be run for service rather than for profit. We need to somehow get back to hospitals run for service. We also need to have health facilities in hospitals such as pleasant exercise opportunities, healthy food, loving care, and an atmosphere free from stress. Family and friends are essential for sick people. Extensive libraries of books, music, and videos can help more than the currently used banal and nerve-wracking television. People need peace to heal.

THE POWER OF THE MIND IN HEALTH

There is a psychological gap between doctors and their patients. This is partly caused by all of the technological machines. The technical jargon of the doctor also widens this gap. Scientific detachment has created a cold, impersonal feeling surrounding some doctors. Doctors can provide co-operation and information during this difficult time for the patient. It is hard for a patient to have dignity when the patient is treated like a malfunctioning machine. The patient is in the doctor's territory and is often terrified. The human body has long been held to be sacred. However, in a doctor's office or hospital, your body is no longer sacred or even your own. It can be cut open for incomprehensible reasons.

Our medical system and hospitals need to support and reassure patients. They should mobilize the recuperative powers of the patient. They should quiet the anxieties of the patient so that the immune system can get to work with full force. Sometimes patients are treated as if the mind and body were completely separate. The psychological assault of a terrible prognosis lowers the patient's expectations and ability to heal. Our bodies follow our minds so that visualization of a positive outcome is a powerful force in healing.

People need techniques to help them cope with disease, impairment, and death. Some people cope using courage, self-control, and perseverance. Others use patience, resignation, and meekness. Still others use duty, prayer, or compassion. With these tools, pain can be more easily borne with dignity. Skill in the art of suffering is becoming a lost art. Please also remember that pain is experienced in different ways by different people even if the location and severity is the same.

Family is important for all kinds of support, but is important especially in transition events like birth and death. The quiet privacy of a home birth is a warm welcome into the family.

Chapter 10

Corporate Science

The modern medical doctor is a scientist in a very unscientific subject. Our culture has an over-enthusiatic, almost religious awe of science and technology. The excellent work done with scientific techniques in hospital emergency rooms are like miracles.

Science depends upon certain fundamental principles. One of these principles is that a certain experiment can be exactly duplicated with the exact same results. Another principle is that all factors can be controlled. A scientific experiment must be held under controlled conditions.

It is impossible to conduct a completely controlled experiment with human beings. The internal environment is never quite the same at two different times—even in the same person, and external factors such as food and exercise taken before the experiment are unique. Air quality and interpersonal factors are different from moment to moment. The electronic environment and bacteria levels are different. Most of all, the power of the mind controls many physiological systems.

Many techniques have been used to compensate for these influences. Science has tried hard to overcome these problems. To a certain extent statistical interpretation of large populations can be made accurate. However, there is no way that any study of human beings can be totally controlled or repeatable. This is certainly demonstrated by the many different and contradictory medical studies.

There are many reasons why scientific studies of drug safety are unreliable. One reason is that most drug studies are done using lab animals. Unlike many people, the lab animals are fed all of the known nutrients in the right amounts and are in good health. The animals are isolated from all chemicals intentionally to test only one chemical. But people are exposed to dozens of chemicals every day through their food, water, air, and skin. The animals are given a larger than normal dose of the drug but for a shorter time than people would take it. Many animal tests only last a few weeks. The effects of consuming smaller doses of the drug for years can only be surmised.

Another reason that scientific testing may not be accurate is that many chemicals can be transformed during processing or in combination with other chemicals, sometimes turning into cancer-causing chemicals. Some chemicals like saccharine were tested and found to be safe from a standpoint of immediate toxicity, but were found to cause cancer over the long term. These delayed effects are difficult to find. They are often found only after widespread use of a drug.

The lack of double-blind studies is cited as the reason that so many therapies outside of modern medicine are invalid. Yet double-blind studies approved Thalidomide, Halcion, and hosts of other dangerous drugs. One way that double-blind studies can be inaccurate is when test subjects are dropped from a study because of unfavorable reactions. For example, if too many people are dropped from a study of a psychoactive drug, the results may look unfairly favorable. Examples of dangerous drugs approved with double-blind studies could fill a book.[1] If double-blind studies are so good, then why are all of these harmful drugs approved?

It is not feasible to certify a drug as safe. It would take too much time and money, and it would take unbiased testing. To get more accurate controls, each age group must be separately tested; then each of those in different stress patterns or with different nutrition patterns.[2] Many other variable factors need to be controlled. To get really tight control would involve a huge number of tests over a long period of time. This is just not feasible.

Modern medicine demands positive proof that therapies work. This is how it rules out most natural healing approaches. However, there are so many contributing causes to any chronic disease that science can almost never isolate a specific cause; look at the difficulty science had proving that cigarettes cause cancer.

Medicinal plants, for instance, have too many constituents to be simple enough to be scientifically tested. With homeopathic treatments, even when double-blind tests show their effectiveness, science rejects them for lack of an acceptable theory of action.[3] This is hardly objective.

The double-blind approach denies that people have any influence on their own healing process. The subjects of the study are held passive, powerless, and helpless. The medical approach is that things are done to people. The natural healing approach is that people are helped to get well and are active participants in that recovery.

BOUGHT SCIENCE

There may have once been a time when no scientist would consider falsifying or slanting results to keep his or her job. Certainly there are still many excellent and unbiased scientific researchers today. However, an increasing number of research scientists now work for corporations and other commercial institutions. Their grants may now depend upon their results.

Some studies of drugs, industrial chemicals, and pesticides are manipulated to get the results that industry wants.[4] Many experimental medical research scientists derive their funding from corporate sources. Many government-funded studies are guided by industry. Additionally, most commercial testing laboratories are run for profit. In order for these corporate labs to receive continuing business, they need to find results that favor the businesses that employ these labs. Doctors can sometimes be dependant on results of drug testing that may have been falsified for money, power, or recognition. Doctors and patients would be wise not to accept drug test results without scrutiny. The funding behind each drug test must be analyzed.

Four researchers working on a study of calcium channel blockers, which are frequently prescribed for high blood pressure, quit in protest after their sponsor removed parts of a draft manuscript describing the drugs' potential dangers such as stroke and heart failure. The source of funding does make a difference. When studies of cancer drugs are conducted by nonprofit institutions they are eight times more likely to find unfavorable conclusions than when they are funded by drug companies.[5]

In one study of 800 scientific journal articles, it was found that almost 300 of the authors had a significant financial interest in the reports. Yet, in none of these studies was the reader informed of the conflict of interest. In a larger study of 62,000 articles, it was found that corporate financial ties were divulged in only 310 of these articles.[6] This makes it difficult to ascertain if bias is present. Industries frequently form nonprofit companies to fund studies so that any conflict of interest is not apparent.

The manufacturer of an anti-arthritis drug, naproxen, was reported to have falsified records of tumors and animal deaths during the safety tests for the drug prior to 1983.[7] It will take the government a long time and it will be a tedious process to remove this drug from the market (naproxen is still being sold as of 2004). The FDA is not as effective in regulating drug safety as we would wish.

When drugs are found to have serious new side effects, they are not normally taken off the market. Only about one percent of drugs are withdrawn from the market.[8] Even severe or fatal side effects of drugs will not usually result in a drug being withdrawn. Instead, a new warning is added to the label of the drug. We must be very careful to read these label warnings because some very dangerous drugs are allowed to remain on the market.[9]

Another example of corporate bias in testing is Industrial Bio-Test Labs. This was a large laboratory that tested thousands of pesticides, drugs, and food additives—about thirty-five percent of all toxicology tests done in America for many years. Based on this company's tests, over ten thousand studies were done to register products for the American market. The United States Environmental Protection Agency (EPA) checked the tests done by Industrial Bio-Test Labs on 200 pesticides. The EPA found that seventy-five percent of these tests were worthless.[10] The officers of the lab were accused of falsifying research to make cancer-causing chemicals appear safe. Reports state that dead rats were surreptitiously replaced, that records were shredded, and that some research was simply fabricated.[11]

The falsely tested pesticides, drugs, and food additives remained on the market. The enormous profits of the pesticide, drug, and food industries continue. This is an unusual case, not because there was fraud, but because it was discovered. Our doctors cannot assume that all pesticides, drugs, and food additives are safe and without health hazards. Any doctor or patient can check the research literature and find dozens of studies showing the dangers of some of the supposedly safe drugs and chemicals.

The corporations that sell medical drugs do the testing of their own drugs. Talk about the wolf guarding the sheep. Naturally, the scientists working for the drug companies are under pressure to find positive results, especially for their own drug inventions. In theory, the FDA examines the testing for validity. In reality, the test results that the FDA looks at may be slanted by the same companies that need to make money on the drugs.

It is not just new drug testing that is under pressure to skew results. In examining the research on menopause, another interesting phenomenon is apparent. The only studies on evening primrose oil listed in the National Library of Medicine database (Medline) "proved" the ineffectiveness of evening primrose oil. It is interesting when drug companies pay for research that tries to discredit natural therapies. This kind of science can be called "bought science." As a result of this negative research, some doctors have assumed that Hormone Replacement Therapy is the only treatment for menopausal symptoms. Recent research shows that Hormone Replacement Therapy is very dangerous.

The testing of cellular telephones and their role in brain tumors is another example of "corporate science." One of the main tests was funded by twenty-five million dollars from a consortium of cellular phone corporations called the Wireless Technology Research Group. These funds came from the same companies who stood to gain financially from the expanded use of cellular telephones. Dr. George Carlo headed this study. He found that there might be a link between these frequencies and genetic damage and cancer. Dr. Carlo has been quoted as feeling that the companies are trying to discredit him because he did not prove cellular phones to be safe.[12] The research on cellular phones and brain tumors is extensive and contradictory. The only conclusion is that these phones have not been proven safe. Any research showing the hazards of cellular telephones will most likely be quickly repudiated by widely publicized and heavily funded corporate research.

When a study finds a problem with an accepted drug, it is not uncommon for the medical journals to run many articles refuting the problems. When a researcher found that a popular vaccination (measles/mumps/rubella vaccine) might contribute to childhood autism, he was harshly criticized in scientific articles.[13] Funding is abundant to support science that defends commercially profitable drugs. Funding is hard to find for studies criticizing drugs. Peer-reviewed journals are also more likely to publish articles that support drug sales.

Another example of corporate science is a study done by the United States Environmental Protection Agency on the components of sugarcane smoke in Hawaii.[14] The result was a report with so much scientific "technospeak" that it was virtually unreadable by most people. A careful study of the report revealed that sugarcane smoke did contain several pesticides in measurable quantities.

Many tricks were used to make the sugarcane smoke appear safe. Instead of reporting the difference in pesticide levels between clean air and sugarcane smoke, the scientists reported the difference between contaminated air and sugar cane smoke. The contaminated air came from fields that already contained pesticides in the air. These scientists then subtracted the amount of pesticides in the contaminated air from the amount of pesticides in the sugarcane smoke to make the sugarcane smoke look safer. Another way that they made the sugarcane smoke look better was to neglect to test for the herbicide *glyphosine*, which is the last herbicide to be sprayed on the sugar cane before the burning.

A clever trick was used to hide the real findings of the report. A one-page cover letter was attached to the front of the report. This letter cleverly masked any findings that might reduce the profits of the sugar or pesticide industries. This cover letter neglected to mention the discovery of chemicals that are formed when pesticides are burned. The cover letter also mentions only two of the three pesticides found in the smoke. Most doctors and politicians were too busy to read the whole report and concluded that sugar cane smoke is safe. These are some of the clever techniques of corporate science.

Corporate science affects doctors. Instead of scientific proof of how safe certain drugs are, doctors sometimes read convenient and profitable lies. The illusion of a firm scientific paradigm also may lead doctors to discount vast areas of knowledge that lack current American scientific verification.

We should always check the source of funding to determine the economic pressures on the scientists. We should look closely at research that proves that a profitable industry is safe. Corporate cover-ups, for example when the tobacco industry hid the bad effects of cigarettes, are more the rule than the exception.[15]

EMPIRICAL SCIENCE

There is another kind of science besides the theoretical, experimental science that supports modern medicine. Empirical science is the science of observation of living systems. This science of observation is used by most of the traditional healing systems worldwide. Throughout hundreds or thousands of years of observation, certain techniques of healing have become proven empirically. In some ways it is not as exact as modern experimental science. However, as we have seen, modern experimental results are often inconsistent or manipulated.

The empirical approach to living systems makes sense. With this approach, it is possible to look at an ill person in his or her environment. It is possible to make use of cultural memory and historical information. The observational approach is how animals verify their instinctual choices of plants to help them heal. In fact, almost all systems of healing are based on this approach except modern experimental science.

Ayurvedic healing, traditional Chinese medicine, chiropractic techniques, homeopathy, and medicinal plant healing are all based upon observation more than experimentation. Over time, these traditional healing systems have found which remedies and techniques work. These healing systems can also look at individual differences between people with the same disease and tailor the medication or treatment.

THE POLITICS OF INFORMATION

A few years ago, there was a harmless and effective mood-enhancing sleeping aid. Tryptophan was sold in health food stores. It is an amino acid, a component of protein. Abundant in milk, it is one of the reasons that milk is relaxing. It is also cheap to produce. It started to become a major seller for the health food industry as a mood-enhancer and sleeping aid for fifteen million people.

The problem with tryptophan in the eyes of the pharmaceutical industry is that it can't be patented. Sleeping aids and mood-enhancers contribute mightily to the profits of this industry. With the growing popularity and availability of tryptophan, the pharmaceutical industry stood to lose millions of dollars.

The then new SSRI drugs like Prozac effectively increased the serotonin levels in the brain. Serotonin is made in the brain from tryptophan. Having sufficient amounts of tryptophan helps the brain produce more of this sedating neurotransmitter. Cheap tryptophan was threatening sales of the expensive, profitable SSRI drugs.

Then something happened. A few batches of tryptophan manufactured in Japan were contaminated by toxins from genetically modified bacteria which were used to make this tryptophan.[16] Many people were severely hurt by the contamination and some died. As a result the FDA declared all tryptophan to be too dangerous to sell over the counter in health food stores. It was banned except by prescription despite the fact that no tryptophan manufactured in any other facility showed any problems. The FDA blamed "the dangers inherent in various health fraud schemes" for the tryptophan problem. This protected the then nascent genetically modified food industry as well as the pharmaceutical industry. The fact that genetically modified bacteria caused the toxins in tryptophan production was long hidden from the public.

A gentle sleeping aid without side effects was thus removed from the reach of most people. Competition for profitable SSRI's and sleeping pills was greatly reduced. The consequences of this process are grave. The pharmaceutical industry guides the products that come to our shelves. Our medical system is not motivated to prescribe or recommend safe and cheap remedies.

Dangerous Tests

Medical diagnostic testing is a necessary and useful part of the diagnostic process. However, too many unnecessary and invasive tests are performed on people. There are various reasons for over-testing. One reason is to avoid malpractice suits. Many tests are considered routine and are always ordered. A few doctors may even be investors in labs and send them business.[17]

This over-testing is hard on patients. Over-testing is also one of the factors that is causing the skyrocketing costs of medical care. There are twenty or more tests routinely ordered upon admission to a hospital. Even most perfectly well people cannot pass this battery of tests. Estimates say that up to fifty percent of all tests are unnecessary and of no help to the patient.[18] Even when only one test is needed, a complex of tests is frequently ordered.[19] The hospitals have convenient forms so that the doctor may check off tests. There is a tendency to check off too many tests.[20] Using the correct tests can be a lifesaving medical necessity. However, we must not overuse these tests.

When a study was done to see if doctors understood the dangers of the most common surgeries and tests, one quarter of the doctors were correct, one quarter overestimated the dangers, one quarter underestimated the dangers, and the rest did not know the dangers.[21]

There are often dangers in invasive testing. One example

of this is the barium x-ray. In this test, barium sulfate is fed to the patient or administered as an enema. After the barium has moved to the area of the intestines to be tested, an x-ray is taken. These x-rays clearly show all of the convolutions and side pockets of the intestines and colon. These are also

How to have Better Lab Tests

Confirm important tests with another lab
Look up the test in a book or website
Know which values are marginal
Use common sense in interpreting results
Normal numbers might not be optimal numbers
Do not take tests merely for research or training purposes
Don't take tests that are unnecessary
In doctor's office labs, check for qualified personnel

the x-rays with the highest radiation exposure of all types of x-rays for patients.

The problem with this procedure comes after the test. It is the nature of bowel pockets to trap food components. The trapped barium chalk is a poisonous substance.[22] With the low fiber diet of most Americans, the irritating and poisonous chalk can stay in the colon long enough to cause trouble. And, of course, the very reason for the barium test is to find vulnerable, damaged tissue in the first place. These barium enemas are very common. However, barium enemas should not be ordered unless absolutely necessary. It is good practice to use gentle laxatives and a change of diet to get rid of the barium. A follow-up low-intensity x-ray to check for residual barium is also a good idea in some cases.

There are safer ways to diagnose and help colon problems. Dietary change towards more laxative foods and less constipating foods might alleviate the problem. Something as simple as a greater intake of clean water may help. Enemas or colonic irrigation may help with blockages or sluggish elimination. Gentle massage and exercise can help move things along. Gentle plant laxatives can be tested for relief. If these natural approaches do not give relief, then progressively stronger treatments and diagnostic procedures can be attempted.

Medical testing is based upon quantitative scales. By relying exclusively on the numbers found in the test results, medical testing often finds problems that don't exist. There will always be someone at the top or bottom five percent of a testing scale. These people need not be labeled abnormal.

When your blood pressure is tested, you may go home with damaging medication even if you don't need it. We should take into account factors that raise blood pressure such as doctor's offices and hospitals. Blood pressure cuffs are almost never recalibrated.[23] Some of the consumer blood pressure devices are not accurate either.

Electronic monitoring machines are not infallible either. We have such faith in machines. EEG (measures brain activity), EKG (heart muscle activity), and x-rays are all subject to poorly calibrated machines and poorly interpreted results. One test of how well doctors interpreted EKGs showed disappointing results. These doctors missed noticing a heart attack on an EKG over twenty percent of the time.[24] This is in proven cases of heart attacks.

X-Rays

X-rays are miracles that allow us to see inside a living person. The various types of imaging used today save lives and help thousands of people. However, there are well-documented dangers to ionizing radiation. X-rays cause thou-

Good X-Rays

Take only medically necessary x-rays
Use lead shielding on adjacent areas
Use only a recently calibrated machine
Make sure that the beam size is as small as possible
Ask the technician not to fill up the film if unnecessary
Have the radiologist study the film for at least 5 minutes
Have the radiologist meet the patient and check his chart

sands of deaths every year, mostly from tumors and cancer.[25] X-rays are a powerful form of ionizing radiation. Ionizing radiation knocks electrons out of their orbits around atoms deep inside our bodies. These high-energy electrons cause a cascade of electrons that leave our biological molecules in a disturbed state. These disturbed biological molecules cause chemical reactions not possible without x-rays. Chromosome damage is common with x-rays.

There is no safe or acceptable dose of ionizing radiation. Even a single radioactive particle can produce permanent mutation in a cell's genetic molecules; this can be the start of cancer. Also, the damaging effects are cumulative as more x-rays are taken. There is no scientific doubt that ionizing radiation such as x-rays cause cancer. Ionizing radiation is far and away the most consistent agent that we know of that causes almost every type of cancer.

We don't need to give up all x-rays. However, we should be using the absolute minimum number required. There were 350 million medical and dental x-rays taken in 2001.[26] With a disease like cancer there are many different factors that contribute to the cause of the disease. Cancer-causing chemicals, smoking, and lack of nutrients all contribute to the causation of cancer. Medical diagnostic procedures that use ionizing radiation such as x-rays also greatly increase the number of cases of cancer, especially amoung younger people and children.

Diagnostic x-rays will be a contributing cause of over two million cancers in a single generation.[27] Ionizing radiation from medical tests such as x-rays is one of the most important contributing factors in cancer causation.[28] Other medical tests that inflict ionizing radiation include computed tomography (CT) scans, mammograms, and fluoroscopy. There has been some progress in lowering the amount of radiation in these procedures. Once ionizing radiation is better recognized as a serious danger by medicine, more steps can be taken to lower dosages and use fewer x-rays. Doctors face a difficult ethical decision if an x-ray is required only for malpractice prevention.

In one study, one third of the x-ray machines were giving off too much radiation and needed repair.[29] The amount of radiation may vary up to 100 fold for the same x-ray in different facilities.[30] In half the cases the x-ray beam is larger than the film.[31] Technicians often increase the size of the x-ray beam to fill the film when it is unnecessary to fill the whole film. These poorly calibrated machines and bad techniques cause unnecessary exposure of the organs and chromosomes. Outside of cigarette smoking, cancer-causing chemicals, and possibly overexposure to sun, nothing causes more cancer than excessive x-ray dosage.[32] Doctors can insist that their patients go to x-ray facilities that are checked and adjusted regularly.

When x-rays are needed and taken, they should be carefully interpreted. Yet it is not uncommon for radiologists to disagree on what these x-rays mean or miss important findings.[33] It is best when a radiologist studies x-rays carefully for several minutes, looks at the patient history, consults with the doctor, and meets the patient. This rarely happens because these hundreds of millions of x-rays are considered routine. X-rays should only be used when needed.

TESTING LABS

Testing laboratories that analyze samples from people can be unreliable. Lab tests are sometimes wrong. It is best to use reliable labs and get important results confirmed by another lab. If important results are not confirmed by a doctor, the patients should get them confirmed. Many tests such as blood counts, urine analyses, tuberculin tests, and chest x-rays are hard to interpret. Even on the common Pap smear, labs consider a thirty percent mistake rate as acceptable.[34] A ninety-five percent accuracy rate on Pap smears could be achieved if doctors and lab technicians did their job with excellence. It is not hard for patients to get information on any lab test. Become an expert on any test important to your health. Bookstores, the Internet, and libraries have information about normal test scores and interpreting results. Most doctors use common sense and their own senses to supplement and verify lab results.

Each testing lab sets its own levels for "normal" for many

tests. For instance, a hospital may test the doctors and nurses to establish a "normal" level for each test. Nevertheless, these levels may be way off from what is optimal or even average for Americans. There are no national norms for many test results.[35] A skewed norm can lead to misdiagnosis. A lifetime of unnecessary treatment and procedures can follow a bad diagnosis.

This raises the interesting difference between "average" and "normal." If we use average cholesterol as a guide in America, we are not using a good target number. Average weight is also not a desirable number. It is best to aim for optimum results rather than just normal or average.

One of the dangers of getting tested is that the test may be done for reasons other than your health. Resident doctors need to do a certain number of procedures to become accredited. For instance, residents may be required to do a certain number of *cytoscopies* per year. Cytoscopies look in the bladder with a flexible tube. This procedure is great if it is needed. It does have dangers and should be avoided if not necessary.

Unnecessary cardiac catheterizations are also dangerous because of the high x-ray dose and possible vascular damage.[36] Be cautious with teaching or research hospitals for these reasons. Make sure dangerous or invasive tests are really necessary for *your* health.

Doctors are putting small testing labs in their offices or group practices in increasing numbers. There are about four times as many of these doctor office labs than hospital and independent labs combined. Quicker results and less transport of the samples are the benefit. The doctor benefits from the extra income. There could be a conflict of interest when a doctor chooses how many tests to perform in his or her own lab. These labs are largely exempt from regulations and may have higher error rates.[37] One study showed that some of these labs had untrained personnel in control.[38] We can keep health care costs down and make medicine safer if we use just the lab tests and x-rays that are truly needed.

Chapter 11

Expanding Our Choices

O ur medical system concentrates on drugs and technological methods and is intolerant of anything perceived as nonmedical. Doctors are convinced in medical school and with journal articles that their way is the only way to treat disease. Our medical system is slow to realize that therapies and approaches outside normal medicine are also needed.

Our medical system could benefit from a better understanding of alternate and complementary methods of healing. Everything done outside of an approved clinic should not be automatically named quackery. Why should it be a problem if grandma or an herbalist helps to effectively heal a minor health problem? Health fraud certainly exists, but we must distinguish between fraud and nonfraud, rather than between medicine and complementary approaches. A restricted view of healing techniques does not serve the needs of patients.

We like to feel that medical professionals are compassionate and respectful. We like to feel that doctors are devoted to healing. On the other hand, any trace of arrogance is a barrier to communication. Sometimes patients feel as if their doctors tell them what to do without listening. In one study, the average time a doctor listened before interrupting the patients was eighteen seconds.[1] No one wants to be treated as a child incapable of understanding his or her own condition or the cure.[2] Patients have emotions, minds, and lives in addition to their symptoms.

Part of the problem is that many people are afraid to make their own medical decisions. They have been conditioned to believe that medical reports and studies are beyond their ability to comprehend. Doctors can encourage patients to learn about their conditions.

Doctors should allow more time for an assessment of the causes of the health problem.[3] It is important for the doctor to educate the patient as to how to prevent a recurrence of the health problem. It takes time for the patient to make important decisions. It also takes time to discuss treatment options, especially alternative treatments that may be safer. We need more than a short chat ending in a prescription or a referral.

People seek medical care when they are scared and need help. Compassionate doctors have respect for their patients and care about their fate. Doctors should also help their patients get copies of their medical records. Otherwise, the patient is unlikely to get the complete records quickly.[4] When a patient shows up with a list of questions, the doctor may think him a bit odd.[5] Nevertheless, a list is a thoughtful way to organize questions and to maximize use of a doctor's time.

Doctors are taught that they get paid for doing, not talking. They see their job as finding something wrong and doing something about it. Doctors too often put the patient on a course of therapy instead of waiting and seeing. This is "Rambo" medicine where the doctor is the hero. Patients, too, expect instant results. Natural healing usually takes a bit of time. Some patients will prefer a slower pace of heal-

A Good Doctor

Is interested in nonmedical approaches
Gives compassionate, respectful service
Is not narrow-minded
Knows he is not omnipotent
Should not be arrogant or contemptuous
Should involve the patient with decisions
Should spend enough time with patients
Should know about alternative remedies
Should explain in plain language
Should let nature heal if there is time

ing if it is permanent and without side effects.

This insistence on instant results is one reason why nondrug options are seldom suggested. Perhaps this concentration on instant results is also why there is so little of health and healing in medical schools and in hospitals. Supportive, nurturing home therapies are not usually discussed because the cure is less instant and dramatic. Our doctors have been listening to the advertisements of the drug companies. They want to give a miracle pill.

Medicine has a vast amount of constantly updated information. There is no way to stay up on all the current medical information. There are very few certainties in how to treat a patient. There is, however, a common façade of absolute certainty. If a doctor cannot help you the doctor may say, "nothing more can be done." This is always wrong.

SUPERFLUOUS SURGERY

The skills of surgery in a modern emergency room are wonderful. Using surgery for chronic diseases means that our medical system has failed to use enough prevention. With these chronic diseases, it is best not to let patients get so unhealthy that surgery is needed. There was a class of doctors in China who were paid only while their patient was healthy. If their patient was sick, these Chinese doctors would need to restore health to get paid again.

Estimates of unnecessary surgery in America range from fifteen percent to twenty-five percent.[6] A Congressional Subcommittee report indicates that 2.4 million surgeries per year are unnecessary.[7] These unneeded surgeries result in a loss of 12,000 lives and four billion dollars.[8] Lives are not the only loss. Surgery is highly traumatic. Additionally, there are over 10,000 people per year dying of anesthesia administration,[9] most of which are preventable.[10] One of the best ways to prevent anesthesia deaths is to require an anesthesiologist to be present during the operation—this is not always required now.

Surgery has a business aspect where sales of the product are the goal. Nonsurgical treatments are less understood by surgeons and mean less money for the surgeons. As the number of surgeons rises, the number of operations seems to grow to keep them busy.[11] A quarter of the one million yearly cataract lens implants may be unnecessary.[12] Many surgeries are also carried out for training or research purposes. Undergoing surgery when it is not necessary is a waste of lives and money.

Hysterectomies are sometimes recommended for problems that can be resolved in a variety of other ways. About 550,000 hysterectomies are performed each year. By age sixty, one in four women will have had a hysterectomy.[13] Only ten percent of hysterectomies have been found to stand up to a second opinion.[14] Rarely is a hysterectomy needed with a woman under forty.

Tonsillectomies are the most common major surgery for children. Almost half a million tonsillectomies are done each year at a cost of half a billion dollars.[15] This operation is rarely necessary, only if the swollen tonsils are actually choking the child. Instead of finding out why the tonsils are swollen, our surgical factories are glad to take them out. Besides the possibility of death and serious complications, the child's immune mechanisms are weakened from the loss of the tonsils. The tonsils are one of the first lines of defense in the body's immune system. It is wrong to assume that tonsils, or any other part of the body, are disposable and unnecessary.

When undergoing a tonsillectomy, children are separated from their family, incarcerated in the hospital, and introduced to the impersonal handling of the medical machine. While tonsillectomies are rarely needed, circumcisions are never medically needed. What a welcome to the world: an unanesthetized circumcision. There are 1.5 million circumcisions performed each year in the US—about eighty percent of male newborns.[16] Routine circumcisions at birth have never been proven to be of any benefit.

Childbirth is another area where unnecessary surgery is common. Episiotomies are not always needed and should not be automatically done. Midwives don't seem to need them. Maybe that is because they work with the mother to ease the child out and use special herbal oils. The surgical delivery of babies by Cesarean section has become all too common. In some hospitals they account for up to twenty-

Unnecessary Surgery

Almost four million unnecessary surgeries are done each year:

250,000 unnecessary cataract lens implants are done yearly
500,000 unnecessary hysterectomies are done yearly
1,000,000 unnecessary tonsillectomies are done yearly
1,500,000 unnecessary circumcisions are done yearly
500,000 unnecessary Cesarean Sections are done yearly

five percent of all deliveries.[17] Over twenty-one percent of births nationwide are now cesarean.[18] Over 900,000 cesarean sections were done in a recent year.[19] Half of these cesarean operations were found to be unnecessary.[20]

Postoperative complications occur in half of all women with Cesareans. This is twenty-six times the rate of complications with normal delivery.[21] One cause of the increase of Cesarean sections is forced delivery. This can be done with drugs or surgery to speed delivery for reasons other than for the health of the child or mother. Another cause of complications is fetal monitoring, especially when electrodes are screwed into the fetus's head. It is best when doctors will work with knowledgeable midwives in home deliveries.

Coronary bypass surgery may also be of little benefit in

some situations. Dietary fat reduction, antioxidant therapy, and careful exercise will improve all of the arteries. Bypass surgery only helps the worst four inches of the arteries. When surgery is really needed, it is a miracle. However, something must be done for the other ninety-nine percent of the arteries. Up to a third of coronary bypass operations may be unnecessary. A seven-year study by the Veterans Administration found that the coronary bypass operation provided no benefit in the vast majority of cases with angina patients.[22]

Surgery is sometimes the wrong way to deal with cancer. The possibility of releasing cancer cells into circulation is one problem. The best way to deal with cancer is to not get it in the first place. The best way to not get cancer is to avoid carcinogens and to build super health. If there is a cancer present, it is vital to avoid carcinogens and build your health and nutrient levels to combat it. This must be done before it is too late. There are many natural therapies for fighting cancer including laetrile, autolysis, antioxidants, cleansing, and medicinal plant therapies that can be customized for each situation. A complete natural program is needed. This natural program may need to be supplemented with surgery or other medical techniques.

The best surgeons are sympathetic and take time with their patients. They care about the person undergoing the surgery as well as the mechanical aspects of the operation.[23] There is more to surgery than just repair and maintenance of the human machine. A great surgeon explains carefully what is going on. It is important for the surgeon to implant positive expectations for the patient's emotional and physical recovery. Major surgery is one of the scariest things that people undergo; a little reassurance is needed.

If you are scheduled for surgery, be sure to get a second opinion from a doctor in a different group. Also try for a less radical surgery. Find a doctor who has a good success rate with this particular operation. Find out the doctor's death rate or complication rate for this operation. Look for an alternative treatment. Nourish yourself before and after the operation with vitamins, minerals, and food—you can do better than regular hospital food. After the operation you had better use preventive measures to keep from needing the surgery again or you will be a foolish patient.

MEDICAL MONOPOLY

One of the most dangerous things about our medical system is that it often denies the effectiveness of any treatment that it doesn't use. Modern medicine claims the exclusive right to treat you even if the origin of the disease is unknown, the prognosis is bad, and the treatment is ineffective. Information from all other cultures seems to be ignored. Instead of learning from other cultures, modern medicine colonizes these cultures to form new markets for pharmaceuticals and medical devices. All knowledge of health and healing from centuries prior to this one is ignored. Even the poor record in healing chronic diseases such as cancer has not convinced our medical experts to look at other approaches.

People put their faith in our medical system. They say, "You fix it, Doc. Do your magic." People give up their control over their own health. With the wonderful technology and all those big words, how can the average person understand medical magic? Nevertheless, we should each take responsibility for our own health. This includes questioning each procedure and therapy.

Medical scientists indicate that mom and grandma are

not to be trusted with our health. They tell us that the medical approach is the only safe approach to take. Once in a doctor's office or hospital, the patient is isolated from the wisdom of friends and family. Today's medicine denies all

---

Surgery Checklist

Look for alternative treatments.
Get a second opinion from a nonsurgeon.
Try for a less radical surgery.
Find a surgeon who is expert in this operation.
What is the success rate for this operation?
What are the complications and how common are they?
Nourish yourself well before the operation.

---

other forms of healing in order to protect itself from economic competition and to protect its pride. Furthermore, it is a crime for others to heal. From blemish to deathly illness, for any health condition, modern medicine has virtually the only license to practice.[24] This lack of competition has resulted in high pay for doctors. Doctors average about $185,000 take-home pay per year while surgeons and specialists take home an average of a quarter of a million dollars per year.[25]

When medical problems are discussed in common language, then treatment and even diagnosis can be within the ability of average people. Many useful therapies can be understood by average people.

Good Doctor, Bad Doctor

How do we know if a particular doctor is a good doctor? Full accountability would help us find the best doctor for the job. For too long, doctors have been regulated only by other doctors. Wouldn't it be nice to know how a doctor did in medical school? It is unlikely that you will see the records. Would you like to know how many malpractice suits were filed against the doctor? It is difficult to find out unless you are a lawyer with plenty of time. Do you wonder if a doctor's license has been suspended? How many times has the doctor done a procedure before? How many deaths occurred? What percentage of the procedures had good outcomes? Has the doctor been in treatment for drug or alcohol abuse? Are crushing debts urging the doctor to order unnecessary tests or surgery? These questions should not be so difficult to answer. However, not even the consumer that has filed a complaint against a doctor can find out the results of the investigation. When malpractice suits are settled, there is a lid placed upon disclosure and publicity. Medical disciplinary sessions are secret. Some of this information is now beginning to be available on the Internet.

Merely being licensed does not assure us that a doctor is still competent.[26] Once a doctor has gotten a state license, the doctor may practice medicine without any competence tests for the rest of his or her life. Competence in specialties is difficult for the patient to ascertain. A doctor may practice any specialty without being certified. That's right; any doctor can practice, say, psychiatry, without any further training.[27] Check to see if your specialist is board certified. An even better way to check if a doctor is a specialist is to see if the doctor has privileges in a hospital in a specific specialty.

Ten states with 20,000 doctors have never had any serious disciplinary action against any doctors, ever.[28] Either these doctors are very well behaved or there is a flaw in the disciplinary system. Even if formal charges are brought against a doctor, the doctor will practice for an average of two and a half years before the case is resolved.[29] In New York there were 2000 backlogged complaints, some for fifteen years.[30] Doctors are discouraged from testifying against other doctors in malpractice cases. In many cases they will lose their own malpractice insurance if they do.[31] Peer reviews almost never punish a doctor for performing unnecessary procedures.[32]

THE EXCLUSION OF ALTERNATIVES

There are two claims that are used to verify that modern medicine is all-powerful: that we live longer because of doctors and that epidemics of infectious diseases were wiped out by doctors. Conspicuous technological therapies are impressive. However, medical treatment is not related to an increase in life expectancy nor is it related to a reduction in our disease burden.[33]

Among thirteen developed countries, America ranks twelfth in life expectancy for teenage boys at age fifteen. We rank tenth in life expectancy for teenage girls at age fifteen.[34] The decisive elements in determining the age that most adults die are nutrition, clean water, and the stability of the population.[35] Even with all of the doctors and hospitals in the United States, the United States ranks all the way down at twenty-eighth in preventing infant mortality.

Technology, along with the doctor, has become almost godlike in medicine. One of the main motivations for seeking medical help is fear. The absolute faith that people have in medicine is both good and bad. It is good when it motivates the recuperative powers of the patient. It is bad when it denies the patient all of the other healing modalities in the world.

Some of the knowledge most threatening to our medical monopoly comes from China. In China it was proven in the late 1960s that ordinary people could use all of the most useful health devices. Within months, thousands of barefoot doctors were trained to use standard medical devices and drugs.[36] Nonprofessional health technicians could now come to the aid of their comrades without the quasi-religious distinction of being a medical doctor.

The other claim that is used to verify that modern medicine is all powerful is that medicine cured the great infectious epidemics. Drugs are portrayed as saviors and miracle workers. For one example, let's take a look at tuberculosis. Tuberculosis was at a peak in 1812 with a seven percent death rate. By the time Koch first isolated the bacillus in 1882 the death rate from tuberculosis had declined to under four percent. The death rate was under two percent when the first sanatorium was opened for tuberculosis in 1910. By the time antibiotics were prescribed in the late 1940s, the death rate was down to less than half of one percent. Tuberculosis was fading away before medicine could come to our rescue.[37]

Typhoid, dysentery, and cholera also had declined before doctors worked out the cause and discovered specific therapies. Nearly all, ninety percent, of the mortality from diphtheria, measles, scarlet fever, and whooping cough was gone before widespread immunizations or antibiotic therapy could have an effect.[38] It was not the doctor with a black bag that cured these epidemics. It was better nutrition, better water, better housing, and sanitation that enabled the resistance of the victims to fight off the infections.

We are grateful that modern medicine has been effective in reducing gonorrhea, pneumonia, and syphilis. Many cases of malaria and typhoid can now be cured quickly. Vaccinations have contributed to the decline of whooping cough and measles and the virtual elimination of polio. But the much-heralded victories over infectious diseases are not matched by successes in chronic diseases.

Today there are new types of epidemics: heart and circulatory disease, cancer, arthritis, diabetes, emphysema, hypertension, obesity, and mental disorders. Modern medicine is failing to prevent or cure these diseases. Survival rates for many cancers have not improved much. Also, more people get cancer every year. Five-year survival rates for all cancers in the United States only increased from forty-nine percent to fifty-four percent from 1974 to 1990.[39] Among people with serious breast cancer, fifty percent do not survive five years, regardless of the medical treatment or lack of it.

Neither can modern medicine be credited with a longer lifespan. Age at death is not related to the proportion of doctors, the number of hospital beds, or to the number of clinical gadgets. Americans live no longer than Europeans and live shorter lives than the Japanese. Also, what we want is more "healthy time," not more time languishing with malingering illness. The medicine of the future that people need and want will be able to give us more of this healthy time.

Thankfully, doctors have been responsible for inventing many of the useful techniques to improve public health. Doctors discovered the value of clean water and sewage treatment, antibacterial procedures, the use of soap and scissors in childbirth, and condoms. These techniques prevent disease.

Control over medicine is placed only in the hands of doctors. This has made it difficult to stop the epidemic of damage from chemical medicine—millions each year are hurt by drugs. There is a growing decline of confidence and trust in our medical system. Doctors have been above criticism because of a traditional reverence given to doctors. In the last century, society has granted medicine the exclusive right to define health and sickness. This is changing, however, as more people take control over their medical treatment.

"Nothing More Can Be Done"

When a doctor tells a patient that "nothing more can be done," this doctor is verbally projecting the death or continuing illness of the patient. This psychological blow to the patient is profound. To reject the effectiveness of all other healing modalities on the planet is an enormous presumption. There are other powers and systems that may save the patient. Neither nature nor the myriads of other healing modalities are even considered when a doctor says that nothing more can be done.

There is always "more that can be done." While specific problems may vary, there are some general principles. It is always a good idea to cleanse the person through the eliminative channels. Nourish the person with whatever is missing. Explore the different exercise options to develop strength. Explore relaxation techniques to aid the immune system. Look at medicinal plants, vitamins, minerals, essential oils, Chinese, and Ayurvedic remedies. Help reduce the impact of some of the major stressors in the person's life such as coffee, alcohol, cigarettes, meat, dairy products, and so on. When these techniques work and healing occurs, we must not just declare it a "spontaneous remission" of the illness. This implies that it was just luck, and it denies the value of these other therapies.

The Secret Language of Doctors

Our medical professionals often use mysterious technical words that prevent people from learning about their own health. This more exact language is fine between doctors where it is more precise than English. However, it is better to use a language that the patient can understand when communicating with the patient. Otherwise, this technical jargon can make patients feel confused.

A doctor with poor communication skills might tell you that you have "gastroenteritis." A better approach is to say, "The lining of your stomach and intestines is inflamed." Using a technical vocabulary is a denial of the patient's ability to understand his or her own body. It is insulting to have technicians use a foreign language in your presence and make judgments about your body as if you were not even there. Perhaps linguistic mystification is a way of making medical decisions unassailable. Even the Catholic Church has long since decided that the mass would be given in the language of the people; it is past time for doctors to speak plainly. It is time to demystify health.

To speak plainly would be to inform the patient of the problem and to invite questions. We need to use familiar vocabulary to experience and discuss our own bodies. There is no reason for a doctor to say "scapula" when the doctor could just as easily say "shoulder blade." Your waiter says, "Your broccoli is underdone" not, "Your cruciferous vegetable has insufficiently agitated molecules." You should insist that your doctors speak plainly to you in the simplest terms.

The Doctor as Teacher

We have somehow had the idea impressed upon us that we are helpless to heal ourselves. Instead of health being just good common sense, medical scientists would have us believe that health is intricate and unfathomable. The belief that self-care is worthless causes much damage. We need to be free from dependence upon modern medicine except for emergencies. We need to learn how to heal, adapt, and help each other. Don't let this dependence on medicine deter you from changing the environment at home or at work if that environment makes you sick. Individuals need to be equipped to understand and deal with illness or impairment. Medical science even makes parents feel impotent to care personally for their kids. We can and must develop the skills and confidence to care for ourselves and for each other.

Our medical system can start teaching when it educates new mothers about safer home delivery and the benefits of breast-feeding. Medical counseling can help teach the family in other ways. Parents and children can be given positive goals to achieve. Our medical professionals should encourage caring, support, and unity within the family.

It would be better if our medical system supported people in self-care rather than trying to control every aspect of peoples' health. We must not continue to make it illegal to care for family and friends. Medicine itself becomes counterproductive when self-care is a felony. Birth, sickness, and death can all take place in the home. We once knew how to handle these situations. We can relearn.

If your doctor is not fit, relaxed, and healthy, then your doctor obviously does not know how to care even for his or her own health. A good doctor is an example to patients of good health habits. When a doctor is overweight or unfit, how can he or she train anyone else in health and the prevention of disease? Our doctors should show us how to live by example.

PART IV

NATURAL THERAPIES

Chapter 12

Choosing Vitamins and Minerals

Despite the fact that much of our food is depleted of vitamins and minerals, some of our medical advisors continue to frown on supplementation. Despite the fact that stressful and polluted American life depletes our body's reserves of vitamins and minerals, nutritional supplements are too easily dismissed by medicine. Despite the vast number of studies showing improved health and disease resistance with supplements, they are rarely recommended. In fact, many doctors even recommend that their patients avoid them.

Vitamins

Doctors, with their training in body chemistry, are in a unique position to learn which supplements can best help their patients fight disease and achieve optimum health.

Vitamin C

Vitamin C has been proven to help our bodies in many ways:

It increases production of antibodies to destroy invading cells.
It inhibits certain carcinogens.
It increases the response of T-cells in our immune system.
It enhances encapsulation of tumors by connective tissue.
It improves the cell-eating ability of the immune system.
It helps protect us from anaphylactic shock.
It enhances the production of interferon.
The list goes on and on.

However, medically prescribed vitamins are likely to be of low quality and not very useful. Medically prescribed supplements usually are synthetic vitamins combined with poorly absorbed minerals. Medical school does not train doctors in the intricacies of supplementing a diet. Only a few medical schools in America include a general nutrition course in the curriculum.[1] It is not normal medical practice to take a diet record and evaluate it to find out which nutrients are needed. Most doctors are too busy keeping up with drug information to learn about the qualities and forms of the vitamins and minerals so that they can properly recommend them. Also, most doctors rely on the government levels of nutrients, which are often too low to help us resist chronic disease or support optimum health.

The best way to get vitamins and minerals is in the diet. Few people have access to organically grown food that is harvested ripe and eaten fresh and unprocessed. This is one reason why supplementation is necessary. The best way to get extra vitamins and minerals is in a carefully balanced multivitamin plus multi-mineral formula. It takes an educated eye to evaluate the amounts and types of vitamins and minerals in a formula.

VITAMIN C

For example, consider vitamin C. A typical medical recommendation is for sixty milligrams of ascorbic acid as a daily supplement. This is the government's average recommended daily intake. Let's take a look at why this is such a poor recommendation. Our bodies need a steady supply of vitamin C for many essential functions. However, ascorbic acid is quickly absorbed and quickly depleted. In fact, if it is given as simple ascorbic acid, the levels of vitamin C in the blood stream actually go down after a short time as widely swinging utilization levels occur. Vitamin C needs to be timed-release and kept at reasonable levels all day and all night. The middle of the night is when dozens of hormones are made, and vitamin C is needed for their synthesis.[2]

Our bodies do not use vitamin C as ascorbic acid directly. In order to be used, the ascorbic acid must first be ascorbated with minerals. *Ascorbation* happens when the

---

Good Vitamin C

Is timed-release
Includes 100 mg of bioflavonoids with
each gram of C
Is ascorbated with mixed minerals
Has a neutral Ph
Is taken in doses ranging from 500 mg to three grams

---

acidic vitamin C is combined with an alkaline mineral such as calcium. This process is forced to occur in the body when vitamin C is taken in the form of ascorbic acid. Much of the ascorbic acid is wasted and the body's needs are less satisfied than if the vitamin C were taken in the ascorbated form in the first place. It is best to take the mixed mineral ascorbated forms of vitamin C. These are ready to go to work in vital areas such as the brain, adrenals, and eyes.

Another problem with ascorbic acid is the acidity. It is similar in acidity to lemon juice. If much is taken, the excessively acidic ascorbic acid can irritate the intestines and kidneys on the way out. There is a need for the ascorbic acid to be buffered to a neutral acidity. Ascorbated vitamin C is already neutral in acidity. Also, let's not forget about bioflavonoids. Bioflavonoids are needed to maintain healthy blood vessel walls. They are found in most plants that naturally contain vitamin C. These bioflavonoids also potentiate the effects of vitamin C as they are part of the vitamin C complex.

Experts on vitamin C recommend at least 500-1000 milligrams daily in a mixed mineral ascorbate form with at least one hundred milligrams of bioflavonoids per 1000 mg of vitamin C. Higher levels of up to 10,000 milligrams daily are needed for active healing. The best forms are ascorbated and timed-release and have added bioflavonoids. Standard medical practice, if vitamin C is recommended at all, is to suggest a mere forty-five to seventy-five milligrams of plain ascorbic acid.

VITAMIN E

Vitamin E is also commonly overlooked by our drug-oriented medical system. Vitamin E is very hard to get in any diet. The modern American diet it is usually low in this vitamin, yet vitamin E is vitally needed in our bodies. One of its important functions is as an antioxidant. Antioxidants scavenge the free radicals that damage arterial walls and cause aging. As an antioxidant, vitamin E also protects blood cells and fat-soluble vitamins.

Vitamin E allows the blood to flow more freely through capillaries. It does this by allowing the blood corpuscles to flow one at a time through capillaries instead of clumping. This is of tremendous importance to the sixty million Americans who suffer from high blood pressure, and this is also why it is helpful in preventing blood clots. Additionally, vitamin E helps scars to heal properly. This is important for skin and blood vessels. It is also essential in cellular respiration and is thus important in preventing cancer. Vitamin E is important for our reproductive system health. There are many more reasons that we all need vitamin E.

Good Vitamin E

Use the natural d form, not the cheap, synthetic dl form
Includes the tocopherols: alpha, beta and gamma
Is taken in doses of at least 200 IU to 400 IU daily

Normal dosage of vitamin E for maintaining good health is 400 IU (International Units) per day; 600 IU for older people. Therapeutic doses range up to 1000 IU's per day. Doses over 400 IU need to be increased slowly, especially when there is high blood pressure. Unfortunately, some medical practitioners either discourage the use of vitamin E or recommend the woefully inadequate twelve to fifteen IU per day of vitamin E that is recommended by the government.

There are several important reasons to find a quality form of vitamin E rather than the synthetic forms found in many supplements. The natural form is in the *d* form (such as d-alpha tocopherol) while the much less useful *dl* form is synthetically made and cheaper. Only nature can make the *d* vitamin E with just the right spin on the molecule. Then there are the tocopherols: alpha, beta, and gamma. These tocopherols potentiate the antioxidant effects. Supplying good quality vitamin E to the body can help in healing hundreds of illnesses.

OTHER IMPORTANT VITAMINS

The best way to get vitamin A is in the form of beta-carotene. A single large raw carrot contains 20,000 IU's of beta-carotene, enough for two days. Generally, any yellow or orange vegetables and roots have good amounts of vitamin A in the form of beta-carotene. These vegetables also have other good nutrients. It is now dangerous to get vitamin A from fish liver oil, as this oil is likely to be polluted. If your multivitamin has vitamin A, it is best if it has only the beta-carotene form and avoids synthetic or fish liver oil forms.

Vitamin D is not really a vitamin. It is not needed to be taken in the diet unless there is zero direct sunlight. Even a few minutes of direct sunlight on just the face will enable your body to make enough vitamin D for the day. It is not the best choice to obtain vitamin D made from irradiated ergosterol in milk or in supplements. A few minutes in the sun each week is preferable.

The B-vitamins used in supplements are almost always synthesized from coal tar. The richest dietary source of B-vitamins is nutritional yeast. This yeast is too bulky to fit inside a vitamin pill. Some vitamin companies sell B-vitamins that are "grown" on yeast or other media. These may be slightly better than the pure synthetic B-vitamins. However, the huge amount of B-vitamins added to so little yeast results in rapid death of the yeast and little assimilation or conversion occurs. If a vitamin has truly natural B-vitamins, it will have a very small amount since not much of this bulky substance will fit into a pill. One solution is to eat plenty of whole grains and add a little nutritional yeast to your diet. If synthetic B-vitamins are added to offset the effects of stress, it is better to take reasonable amounts rather than megadoses.

Each of the other vitamins also plays a role in health and in disease. It is vital to make sure that when a cell needs a vitamin, it is present in the bloodstream. From vitamin A to vitamin U, our health professionals need to know how much and what vitamin forms are desirable to support optimum health. The ideal way to take vitamins is in a carefully balanced formula. Along with the multivitamin and mineral supplement, additional vitamins can be added as needed for special healing needs. This is one of the wonderful ways that we can support the natural healing ability of the body.

There are many vitamins for which there has been no Recommended Daily Allowance (RDA) set. These vitamins are often missing from cheaper multivitamins. Choline and inositol are B-vitamins that are important for our nervous system. Biotin is another needed nutrient and a member of the B-vitamins. It can be made in healthy intestines. Vitamin B-15 in the form of dimethylglycine is helpful for getting oxygen into the energy factories inside the cell (the *mitochondria*). Vitamin B-17 is important in controlling cancer. Also known as amygdalin, it is found in many seeds. Vitamin U is found in cabbage and is very useful in healing skin ulcers and stomach ulcers. Vitamin T is found in sesame seeds and helps control anemic tendencies. Vitamin K is needed for blood clotting; it is found in many vegetables. Sometimes the essential fatty acids are called vitamin F. They are like a vitamin in that they are required in the diet and cannot be made in the body. For too long these important nutrients have been neglected by medical scientists and the U. S. Department of Agriculture.

MINERALS

Minerals in the diet cannot be taken for granted. As a result of chemical farming, only nitrogen, phosphorus, and potassium are routinely added to the soil. All other minerals and trace minerals are being depleted or are already depleted from the soil. When the right minerals are present in the soil, the soil microbes and rootlet fungi prepare them for assimilation into the plants. With chemical farming, the microbes are often not present and the rootlet fungi are not fully functional. Plants can only assimilate the minerals that are in the soil. For example, if there is no zinc in the soil, then there will be no zinc in the plants. Most states have depleted zinc in their agricultural soil.

Dietary minerals can be separated into two types: macro minerals and trace minerals. The macro minerals are needed in quantity all of the time. Calcium and magnesium are examples of macro minerals that are needed in large quantities. Other common macro minerals are phosphorus, potassium, and sodium. A natural diet of vegetables, fruits, whole grains, nuts, and seeds provide all of these minerals—especially if the food is grown organically. However, please note that a healthy organic diet is just what most Americans do not eat.

People are commonly told to get their calcium from dairy products. Calcium is extracted in the stomach with stomach acid. One problem with dairy products is the neutralization of the stomach acid, which interferes with calcium uptake. Another problem with using a dairy product as a calcium supplement is the excess protein present in many dairy products. Excess protein in the diet leaches calcium out of the body.[3] Calcium is abundant and assimilable from brown sesame seeds, other seeds, nuts, beans, and green leafy vegetables.

Even though we need smaller amounts of trace minerals, we need them just as much. There are about seventy trace minerals that we now know to be needed by the human body. Common examples are selenium, zinc, iron, manganese, chromium, molybdenum, germanium, vanadium, and copper. We cannot be optimally healthy and disease resistant if we lack even a single trace mineral. These minerals are all dependent on each other. For proper utilization, all must be available in the body. The key to trace minerals is balance. We need only a few micrograms of copper every day. We need dozens of milligrams of zinc. Too much of any one mineral is unbalancing and interferes with the utilization of the other minerals.

The best way to supplement the diet with trace minerals is to take them all together in a balanced formula. Colloidal trace minerals from ancient seabed deposits are available in tablets or mixed in with multivitamin-mineral supplements. These are well balanced and are easily assimilated. Other trace mineral supplements are also available. Seaweeds are another good source of trace minerals if the seaweeds come from unpolluted oceans. When organic farms use rock dust containing trace minerals to enhance their soil, we can get the trace minerals directly from our food.

ASSIMILATION OF MINERALS

It is important for our health advisors to know which mineral forms are more assimilable and which forms are less assimilable. Minerals must first be digested and absorbed into the intestinal wall cells. The minerals must then be released into the blood and transported to the cells where they are needed. The minerals do us no good unless they are suc-

cessfully delivered across the cell membranes to the tiny or-
ganelles inside the cells.

Elemental minerals like calcium carbonate, iron sulphate,
elemental chromium, or magnesium carbonate are poorly
absorbed and can irritate the intestinal wall. Only one to
nine percent of calcium carbonate is absorbed because it is
not organically bound. Elemental minerals often bind permanently to the commonly found phytate or oxylate molecules in the stomach and are excreted. Minerals must be
bound to organic molecules (a process referred to as chela-
tion) to be properly utilized. Minerals occurring naturally
in food are always bound to organic molecules.

CHELATION AND TRANSPORT OF MINERALS

Certain chelating agents help us to absorb minerals.
Some chelating agents are better than others. The glucon-
ates, citrates, and lactates improve mineral absorption. One
example is iron gluconate. Unfortunately, the acid conditions
in the stomach break some of these chelating bonds, causing some of these minerals once again to become elemental.
However, if the mineral supplements are taken with food,
the amino acids present in the food will chelate with the
free minerals and aid absorption. Some mineral supplements
are already chelated with amino acids. Amino acid chelates
are more resistant to being split up in the stomach and help
transport the minerals into the intestinal cells.

Once a mineral is absorbed from the intestines, it must
be transported to the blood stream and then to the target
cells. A single mineral that has been chelated with glucon-
ates, citrates, lactates, or amino acids may need several car-

rier molecules to be transported to its target cell.

Some minerals such as magnesium can be chelated with aspartic acid. The aspartates are quite efficient. They can transport their minerals to the inner membranes of the target cells. The aspartates have an affinity for liver and heart tissue. In addition to aspartic acid, some minerals are chelated with vitamin C (ascorbic acid). These mineral complexes are called ascorbates. Ascorbates such as calcium ascorbate are good mineral transporters that deliver the minerals directly to the inside of the cell.

Minerals can also be chelated with orotic acid, also known as vitamin B13. This is a very stable chelate that survives stomach acid with little change. The mineral orotates are absorbed intact into the intestinal cells and are released into the bloodstream without needing any secondary carriers. These mineral orotates are then able to be transported across the outer and inner cell membrane and are delivered to the inside of the target cell. Here the orotates can be used immediately inside the cells in metabolic processes. These orotates have a special affinity for bone and cartilage tissue.

We must inspect our mineral supplements carefully to be sure that they are in forms that will make the long journey from our mouths to the inside of our cells. Each mineral must also be taken in just the right amount.

Calcium

It is disappointing to see that most prenatal vitamins have hard-to-absorb minerals. Calcium from such sources as oyster shell, dolomite, and calcium carbonate are very poorly assimilated into our cells. All forms of calcium always depend on magnesium, lysine, and sunshine to be utilized properly in our bodies.

The government recommended levels of 800 milligrams of calcium per day are generally adequate if supplied by the diet or in assimilable forms. In the body, estrogen helps the absorption of calcium. Postmenopausal women need more calcium to keep their bones solid because their natural estrogen levels decline with age. Because of the recently publicized problems with estrogen hormone replacement therapy, we should be encouraging natural estrogen production. This can be assisted with medicinal plants such as black cohosh, panax ginseng, and licorice root. Additionally, exercise helps strengthen bones.

MAGNESIUM

Magnesium is a macro mineral vitally needed by all of our cells. It is best to get it from organic food such as green vegetables. Because it is needed for nerve transmission, it helps us to relax and sleep. Nervousness can be a sign of low magnesium levels. We would be wise to check to see if magnesium will help with nerve problems before considering toxic or addictive drugs. Convulsions and tremors can also be signs of magnesium depletion. This natural tranquilizer is very helpful for depression as well. It is easy to check magnesium levels with a diet record before prescribing Prozac or even St. John's wort. We can become depleted in magnesium from alcohol use, diuretic use, fluoride in water, synthetic vitamin D, and from eating raw vegetables containing oxalic acid (like kale). The ascorbated or amino acid chelated forms are best if magnesium is to be taken in supplement form.

ZINC

One mineral that we should not overlook is zinc. Zinc is an important component of dozens of hormones and enzymes. It is needed by the prostate gland and also to make insulin. Zinc is an important antioxidant that helps prevent arterial damage and aging. It prevents the liver from releasing excessive amounts of vitamin A. It is vital for the immune system. We need zinc to make DNA (Deoxyribonucleic Acid) and RNA (Ribonucleic acid).[4] We must not overlook the fact that zinc is often missing from diets. The best forms of supplemental zinc are zinc picolinate, chelated zinc, ascorbated zinc, or zinc monomethionine. Although the government daily requirements are fifteen milligrams for a man, optimal health can best be achieved by taking sixty milligrams in a high-quality form. Zinc is available in organically grown beans, mushrooms, pecans, seeds, whole grains, and soybeans. This availability, of course, depends on the soil having zinc in the first place. Nutritional yeast is an excellent source of zinc and many other needed nutrients.

Each of the other minerals has an optimum daily amount. Each of these minerals has forms that are best to ensure assimilation into our cells. Make sure that you get a balanced amount of all of the minerals, and you will become more disease resistant and stronger.

Chapter 13

Natural Healing Solutions

Alternative and complementary remedies are remedies that do not fall within the normal scope of practice of a modern medical doctor. These remedies are not normally presented in medical school although elective classes in alternative or complementary medicine are slowly becoming more common.

Throughout the ages, millions of people around the world have used natural remedies and have found these remedies to be effective. Medical science will often discount as "anecdotal evidence" traditional use of a medicinal plant even after thousands of years of success. Medical science seems to believe only in remedies that have been approved by the pharmaceutical industry through the FDA.

It is not enough to merely substitute natural remedies

for drugs and surgery. We need to get out of the "symptom-treat" revolving door. Our current medical system waits for disease to occur before treatment begins. Especially for chronic disease, cure is difficult. We should maintain a health strong enough so that we don't need even these natural remedies.

One type of natural remedy is herbal medicine. Pharmaceutical companies are discovering the profit potential of medicinal plants. Small herb companies are being bought up by multinational drug corporations. Large sums of money are being spent on advertising these medicinal plant remedies. The doctors who ignore the importance of botanical medicine and other forms of complementary healing are being left behind.

These various complementary and alternative remedies are not just new drug-like things to be prescribed like any other medical therapy. There are philosophies behind each type of therapy. The mode of action is rarely to attack germs within the body or to directly regulate internal chemicals. With many natural therapies the action is to help us regain our own ability to maintain an internal balance.

With medicinal plants, one therapeutic action is to supply nutrients such as trace minerals or bioflavonoids. Herbalists have classified medicinal plants into about one thousand property and action categories. Some plants act as a tonic to strengthen tissues. Other plants act as antispasmodics; some are mild like chamomile, while others are extremely powerful like belladonna. Astringent plants contract tissues to expel fluid, clear toxins, and reduce swelling. Other plants stimulate the body's natural defenses or act directly upon pathogens.

There are many therapies that can complement modern medicine. Acupuncture is part of a highly developed and effective Traditional Chinese Medicine. With homeopathic remedies, the body's reaction to the remedy is carefully planned to restore health. Various forms of massage can circulate blood and fluids, relieve nerve pain, adjust posture, relax the person, and heal damage. Topical applications of essential oils can selectively affect just the area that needs healing. These are some of the rich and varied resources outside of the realm of pharmaceutical medicine.

A Painful Example

There are many natural treatment possibilities for a forty-five year old man with recurring migraine headaches. This man had been getting excruciating migraine headaches three times a week for ten years. He went to many doctors and clinics. He felt that he had gone to the best doctors in the world. He had received many drugs. The drugs gave no lasting relief from his headaches and several gave him bad side effects.

His doctors went so far as to try repeated surgeries on his neck. This not only made no improvement, but they wanted to operate again to reverse the last operation. At the time I met him he was on many harsh medications and contemplating suicide. He is a wealthy man with a lovely wife and three young children. He has paid a fortune for his medical treatments. His doctors were starting to tell him that they had done all that could be done. We will discuss some natural and complementary treatment options that his doctors did not suggest.

It seems clear that a stress reduction program could reduce the frequency and severity of the headaches. The first step is to keep a stress record. This record will list the significant stresses during at least one week. Some correlation may even be seen with the migraines. Then a customized program can be developed to reduce the effect of the stressful situations on the man. His migraines were often triggered on the freeway. Car bumper reflections of sunlight could start the agony for him. Wraparound dark glasses with good polarized protection could help with this trigger.

This man needs to have a systematic stress reduction program to keep him from getting tensed up so often. This stress reduction program needs to be personal and unique. For example, if reading the newspaper in the morning gets him uptight, it may be better to take a hot tub instead. A siesta a day could keep the migraines away.

A relaxation program is different than a stress reduction program because it deals with the impact of stresses that cannot be reduced further. Migraines are keyed to tense nerves and also high blood pressure. Relaxation programs lower blood pressure thus relaxing capillaries in the head. Massage, hot tubs, meditation, autogenic relaxation, saunas, swimming, walking, music, gardening, and exercise all can help us to relax. Doctors can have information at hand for these and many more relaxation options. Biofeedback can enable a person to control his blood pressure at will. This can be used to forestall an impending migraine.

Many of this man's migraines happen from 1:30 a.m. to 3 a.m. This is a time when hundreds of hormones are produced in our bodies. Perhaps a diminished level of vitamin C in his blood, a lack of essential fatty acids, or low trace minerals might have been contributing to low hormone production.

We need to see to it that the basic nutrients are available in our blood stream twenty-four hours a day. This man had tried vitamin C but did not use the more effective timed-release, ascorbated formulation. One of his medical prescriptions was testosterone shots. These had only a temporary benefit, and the man did not want the shriveled testicles that this might cause. We should not forget that when a hormone is injected, it causes the production of that hormone by our bodies to drop. This is the wrong direction for us to be going.

There are many types of bodywork that can help with migraines. It might be very helpful to use neuromuscular therapy to remove painful knots in the muscles and connective tissue especially in the head and neck. Shiatsu is a systematic therapy that balances the flow of blood and nerve energy throughout the body. Pressure points are pressed symmetrically all over the body for a complete balancing. Rolfing and other structurally balancing types of bodywork can remove constant strains and pains from a person's life. Specific work around the head can relieve tensions between the skull bones themselves. This man never received any information about any of these excellent massage techniques.

Fitness can have a positive impact on the arterial system. A carefully tailored fitness program should include not only aerobic exercise and strength training, but also rebounding, inversion, walking, and stretching. This fitness program should be targeted at overall health improvement. Overall health improvement is just what our medical system needs to incorporate. As the elasticity of the artery walls is increased, the migraines might improve. Endorphins from regular aerobic workouts will definitely help with the pain.

This migraine sufferer did consider some aspects of food. He systematically left suspected food triggers out of his diet. What he did not do was improve his diet. Each week a bad food should be chosen to reduce. Each week a superfood should be introduced for tasting. Over time junk and polluting foods are reduced and more nutrients are introduced. Coffee and other caffeine-containing beverages can contribute to headaches. It would be wise to experiment with a month of reduced or eliminated caffeine use to see if the headaches decreased. It is likely that the overall health benefits from making these changes will help the migraines. It is also very likely that his risk of cancer, heart attacks, prostrate problems, and digestive disturbances will be reduced from these dietary improvements.

His medical therapy did not include peppermint (*mentha piperita*) oil or other volatile balms rubbed directly on the head. Basil oil, Chamomile oil, Lavender oil (*lavandula angustifolia*), and Eucalyptus oil (*eucalyptus globulus*) are all used in balms to relieve migraines specifically. These give instant relief and a feeling of some control over the pain. Valerian root, lobelia, feverfew (*chrysanthemum parthenium*), ginkgo (*ginkgo biloba*), skullcap, and wood betony (*betonica officinalis*) are all medicinal plants recommended for migraines. He never tried Vitamin B3, phenylalanine, or magnesium. This is despite the fact that these are cheap, safe alternatives to such terrible drugs as prednisone. It is no surprise that his medical treatment did not include the Chinese patent medicine *Chuan Qiong Cha Tiao Wan* used for migraines. *Jatiphaladi churna* is an Ayurvedic remedy used for migraines. Dong quai (*angelica sinensis*) is used in China to lessen migraines. Physicians are not normally trained in homeopathic medicine. Nevertheless, the homeopathic remedy *coffea* has a high likelihood of helping.[1] Future medical care will try these safer and gentler alternatives before polluting a person with potentially toxic and depleting chemicals.

The effect of certain common pesticides (the organophosphates) is to cause spontaneous nerve contractions. This often contributes to epilepsy, multiple sclerosis, and migraines. Storage and use of these pesticides in the home should be considered as a special risk in migraines as well as a general health risk. Electromagnetic stresses should also be considered. A simple meter can check for harmful electric, magnetic, and microwave fields around the home and office. Certain handheld cellular phones expose the user to

Migraine Remedies

- ☐ Stress reduction with naps, hot tubs, meditation, saunas, swimming, walking, music, gardening, and exercise.
- ☐ Biofeedback to control blood pressure.
- ☐ Basic nutrients: natural food plus a multivitamin, vitamin C, essential fatty acids, and trace minerals.
- ☐ Neuromuscular therapy, shiatsu, and body alignment therapies like Rolfing can help tremendously.
- ☐ A balanced fitness program with aerobics, rebounding, inversion, stretching, warm-ups, and walking.
- ☐ Improve the diet with less junk food and more superfoods.
- ☐ Topical balms and essential oils for instant relief: wintergreen oil (*gaultheria procumbens*), basil oil, chamomile oil, lavender oil, Tiger Balm™, and eucalyptus oil (Dilute all except Tiger Balm™ before use).
- ☐ Valerian root, lobelia, feverfew, ginkgo, skullcap, and wood betony are medicinal plants that help migraines.
- ☐ Vitamin B3, phenylalanine, magnesium, the Chinese patent medicine *chuan qiong cha tiao wan*, Ayurvedic *jatiphaladi churna*, the plant *dong quai* and the homeopathic remedy *coffea*.
- ☐ Reducing possible migraine triggers such as pesticides, microwaves, and cell phone use.
- ☐ A cleansing program.

the highest levels of microwaves. Pressing a cellular phone to the head should be considered as a possible aggravating influence on migraines.

Another excellent approach is systematic cleansing. American bodies take in many toxins and are frequently clogged up. This contributes to many problems. Bowel cleansing, liver flushing, skin cleansing, and kidney cleansing are all appropriate for virtually any health problem.

The point is not that these approaches are sure to cure migraines, although it is likely that they might. The problem is that none of these approaches were tried by modern medicine. All of these and more should have been tried before resorting to spinal surgery and prednisone. This approach is to build the health to higher and higher heights until all health problems disappear.

BOTANICAL MEDICINE

Doctors swear an oath to "first of all, do no harm." Find a doctor who has let this principle be a guide in his or her practice. First, in any but an emergency situation, we need to try the gentlest approach. The best gentle approach after basic lifestyle changes is usually a medicinal plant. It is only after exhausting the range of medicinal plants and other gentle therapies that we should resort to chemical drugs with their harsher side effects. It is also best to try these gentler treatments before undergoing surgery if there is time.

Observation and experience through the centuries has given us the correct medicinal plants to use for many health problems. More recently, the plant chemicals have been isolated and identified. The isolated constituents have verified the traditional use of the plants in more and more cases. Additionally, the components of the botanical remedy that are not recognized as active may also play a synergistic role in modifying the effects of the more active substances. Many components such as enzymes defy chemical analysis yet play important roles in the effects of medicinal plants. Medicinal plants are gaining scientific recognition and are undergoing an important revival.

There are many reasons why whole herbal medicines are often superior to pure chemical drugs. The beneficial interactive effects of the constituents of the whole botanical medicines may disappear when only one constituent is used, especially if it is used in a pure, isolated drug form. Easily assimilated forms of minerals play an important role in many botanical remedies. The complex structure of the botanicals normally releases the medicinal components more slowly than pure pharmaceuticals do, thus reducing side effects from rapid assimilation. If you take too much of a botanical it is usually obvious; you might feel queasy or get tired of the bitter taste. This reduces the likelihood of an overdose and guides the dosage. When you take isolated drugs you feel no perceptible immediate indication of overdose until it is too late. The fact is that we have had thousands of years to accustom our bodies to the natural medicinal plants.

A health professional who is educated in medicinal plants will develop a personal rapport with each plant that he uses. One gets to know the plants almost as if they had a personality. Personal experience in using the medicinal plants helps the professional herbalist to understand the plant. It is important to recognize the differences in preparation, use, and effect between leaf, flower, root, and bark. We must learn to distinguish fresh and potent herbal products from stale and worthless ones. It is helpful if our health professionals can tell us how to prepare the plants. Hopefully, our botanical prescriber will have had occasion to at least taste and smell the plant.

Patients also get personal with their medicinal plants. They see the herbal cure as closer to nature and more natural for humans. People often become grateful to a plant that cures their illness. We can sometimes feel a sense of personal empowerment and intention to heal as we prepare these plants for use.

Medicinal Plants are the obvious choice for first treatment before harsher chemicals are used. The gentler of the medicinal plants are especially valuable for long-term therapy where the cumulative side effects of harsher drugs would cause problems. Chronic heart disease, arthritis, high blood pressure, and many other chronic diseases should be treated with these gentler medicinal plants whenever possible.

Medicinal plants, with their gentler side effects, are especially well suited for convalescence and rehabilitation. For degenerative diseases of the heart, hawthorne berries increase cardiac circulation. For arthritis and rheumatic complaints, alfalfa (*medicago sativa*), dandelion root, or burdock root are excellent for long-term corrective treatment. There are hundreds of well-researched medicinal plants to choose between. For comprehensive information on over a thousand of these natural remedies see the computerized database, *Natural Healing Solutions.*[2]

Many people make the mistake of discounting all natural remedies as weak and ineffective. Natural remedies span the entire spectrum from very powerful to gentle enough for a baby. We must not wrongly assume that medicinal plant drugs without toxic effects are worthless. Toxic effects are not necessary for effective healing with medicinal plants.

Foxglove (*digitalis purpurea*)—the source of digitalis, colchicum (*colchicum autumnale*), and belladonna (*atropa belladonna*) are examples of powerful, potentially toxic, and fast-acting plants. Fennel (*foeniculum vulgare*), peppermint, hops (*humulus lupulus*), and hawthorne are examples of gentle and effective medicinal plants. A single stale tea bag of chamomile in a cup of boiling water is surely not much help with a nervous stomach. A cup of tea made with boiling water poured over a quarter of a cup of fresh chamomile flowers and steeped with a cover for five minutes has a potent and

Why Choose Medicinal Plants Over Drugs

- ◻ Slow release of the medicinal components helps reduce unwanted side effects
- ◻ They give natural clues that we are taking too much, like bitterness and nausea
- ◻ They are good for first treatments instead of toxic drugs
- ◻ Plants are great for long-term therapy with chronic disease
- ◻ Plants are closer to nature and more natural for humans
- ◻ They may contain enzymes and assimilable minerals
- ◻ There are synergistic interactive effects between the constituents
- ◻ Some plant components play a role in modifying the effects of the more active substances
- ◻ Toxic effects are not necessary for effective healing with medicinal plants
- ◻ They are perfect for convalescence and rehabilitation
- ◻ Medicinal plants are usually much less expensive than drugs

powerful soothing effect. We must not confuse beverage tea with medicinal plant use.

Herbal medicine should be introduced in premedical and medical school, if not earlier. It can become a specialty for certain doctors. This is not a sideline of medicine, but an integrated study in itself that can benefit the doctor's general knowledge. Many doctors in Europe and around the world understand medicinal plants and incorporate them into their practice on a regular basis.

Herbalists tend to get excited about their favorite medicinal plants. This can lead to rather imaginative lists of ills cured by these plants. Herbalists and pharmacognosists (those who study plant constituents) are sifting through the recorded uses of these plants and finding the best plants for each health problem—and each person. It is one of the challenges and duties of modern science to sift through these historic resources and learn the most effective cures.

One way to do this is through a search for what can be called "cross-cultural convergence." This happens when a medicinal plant is used in different cultures for the same purpose. For instance, passion flower (*passiflora incarnata*) is used for insomnia in Utah, India, Iraq, and Amsterdam, among other places. This leads one to believe that it is not imagination or coincidence that passion flower is helpful with insomnia. The list of verified medicinal plant uses is growing long.

Our scientific medical system tends to think that only double-blind studies have any validity in verifying the action of a drug or botanical medicine. However, if a plant has been used for a long time, is prescribed by many doctors worldwide, and is demanded by patients, then the plant action should be accepted. Doctors also demand, especially in a hospital setting, an instant response to their drugs. But it is this instant response that is causing so many of the side effects from the drugs. Nature heals better if given a little time. Especially in general practice, where many conditions are not life threatening, the less toxic botanicals are much safer and should be widely used.[3]

Even when medicinal plants are carefully tested and found to have powerful effects, most doctors will not prescribe them. As one example, consider a report in the journal *Cancer* on a University of Texas study.[4] This was a study of two Chinese herbs, astragalus (*astragalus membranaceous*) and ligustrum (*ligustrum lucidum*). These two medicinal plants were found capable of aiding immune function in ninety percent of the cancer patients tested. These medicinal plants were also found to provide some protection against the damaging effects of chemotherapy and radiation. Unfortunately, it is not common for cancer experts to recommend them.

It is normal medical practice to use drugs like Zantac and Tagamet to treat stomach ulcers. One alternative is aloe vera juice, which is made from the gel of a cactus. It can give immediate relief from stomach ulcer pain. We should not ignore such a safe, cheap remedy. Aloe vera juice can also be taken after the drugs that increase the incidence of stomach ulcers, such as aspirin and ibuprofen. These drugs slow the production of prostaglandins that assist our stomach lining in secreting mucus. The mucilaginous and soothing aloe vera juice coats this stomach lining while promoting healing. This is one of the many ways that medicinal plants can ameliorate the bad side effects of drugs. Knowledgeable doctors are also now using aloe vera gel in burn centers. Aloe vera gel is certainly an excellent burn remedy for mild burns, especially if the gel is fresh.

Hawthorne berries are safe and have been widely tested for centuries. Hawthorne berry jam is popular in England. These berries have the ability to strengthen the heart and circulatory system. These red berries are principally used for arteriosclerosis, angina, and arrhythmia. Whenever there is weakness in the heart, these friendly berries have a place. They increase the circulation in the heart's coronary arteries, and they dilate the coronary blood vessels. The heart muscle is strengthened and energized. Long-term therapy is safe, cheap, and without bad side effects, although it is contraindicated with ulcers and colitis.

Evening primrose oil has been favorably reviewed in more than 200 European studies and is widely used in European hospitals.[5] It supplies essential fatty acids which act as precursors to hormone production. It is used for easing premenstrual syndrome. It is soothing and nourishing to the nerves, especially to the myelin sheaths of the nerves. This is why it is used for multiple sclerosis, epilepsy, menopause, hot flashes, and nervous conditions. It is a nourishing and safe oil. It is unwise to prescribe drugs with serious side effects when this natural remedy would be effective.

ESSENTIAL OILS

Essential oils are made by distilling oils out of plants. These oils have many of the active principles of the plant in a concentrated form. They can be mixed with massage oils and rubbed directly on the area that needs them. They are potentially dangerous if used internally, so caution is needed for internal use. Even externally they need to be diluted to avoid skin irritation. The smells of the oils are pleasant and affect emotions. Essential oils are also used in ointments, insect repellents, shampoos, soaps, toothpaste, and lotions.

There are over one hundred essential oils in common use. Some of the most widely used essential oils are lavender, rose, peppermint, eucalyptus, chamomile, and orange blossom. Essential oils may be used for a variety of reasons including anti-inflammatory action, painkilling action, antiseptic action, sedative action, and antispasmodic action. They go to work instantly, especially when used for pain. Be aware that there are many oils of poor quality on the market. Cheap oils are sometimes extracted with dangerous solvents and may contain synthetic perfumes. These oils are not suitable for therapeutic use. Properly made rose oil requires 30,000 to 60,000 roses for each ounce of essential oil.[6] Essential oils and aromatherapy are wonderful, effective therapies that could complement many medical therapies.

MASSAGE THERAPIES AND HYDROTHERAPY

A gentle, probing massage is not as common as you might expect at a modern medical clinic. Yet through the ages, healers have been touching people. There are many forms of massage from the gentlest to the deepest. Massage can be used for relaxation, to heal an injury, for diagnosis, for long-term postural changes, or as a method of topical application. You might want to choose a health provider that gives a personal and compassionate touch. It would be helpful for medical practitioners to take continuing education that could teach them about the various techniques of massage. This would help them choose the correct massage techniques for referral. While there is some overlap between physical therapists and massage therapists, no person who has been to both could confuse them.

Touch for diagnosis

Health professionals can learn many things about people when they perform massage. A health history becomes much more useful after massage gives personal knowledge and acquaintance. Is the person too flabby or too tight? Areas of tension indicate where the person may be lifting or working wrong. Is the person too hot or too cool? While a thermometer checks the inside of the body, massage can distinguish many different temperatures on the skin and beneath the skin. Muscle spasms and active healing areas are noticeably hotter than the surrounding areas. Swollen lymph nodes are easily detected. Skin problems are noticed and can be discussed by a massaging health professional.

The ability of a person to relax is a vital necessity in modern life. Checking how long it takes for a person to get to a "relaxation response" gives important information. Sensitivity to pain is apparent with massage. If a person falls asleep during a massage, it is obvious that the person is exhausted. Skin color is a good indicator of circulation. Foul or strange body odors are noticed and can be addressed. Emotional states become clearer from massage and can have a profound effect on health and disease. Massage is an invaluable diagnostic tool that is underutilized in modern medical clinics.

There are many different forms of massage around the world. Swedish massage helps circulate the blood and lymph fluids. It is also good for relaxing muscles and keeping the tendons limber. Shiatsu massage was developed in Japan. This massage methodically moves over the body releasing tension along the spine and the rest of the body. Neuromuscular therapy releases trigger points with finger pressure. It is very effective in healing injuries and relieving pain and tension. Rolfing and other forms of structural massage can help to straighten posture by moving and stretching underlying sheets of fascial tissue. Lomi-Lomi is a Hawaiian form of massage that uses round stones to smooth out muscles. There are many more types of massage that are used in different cultures to heal and relax.

Neuromuscular release

Back injury is one of the most common types of injury in America. Millions of people suffer from chronic back pain. One of the causes of this pain is described as *neuromuscular trigger points.* These trigger points often occur between the muscles and the tendon attachments. The trigger points are

Massage Therapies

Swedish massage for circulation and to relax muscles
Shiatsu to systematically release tension
Neuromuscular therapy for releasing tight spots from old injuries
Structural alignment therapy to straighten you up
Sports massage to prevent and heal injuries
All massage is useful for diagnosis

tense and hard. They are painful to the touch. Trigger points are left over damage from old injuries. They can last for a long time because circulation is limited in these small areas. A practitioner of neuromuscular massage therapy can release these points by finger pressure. It takes close cooperation between the therapist and client. Part of the effect is achieved by using the exhalation of the breath to relax the trigger point. One reason that this works so well is that as the acid content of the blood is reduced through respiration, the ability to release acidic wastes into the bloodstream is heightened.[7] A tremendous amount of relief is felt with this therapy. The results are permanent unless the damage is repeated. Without this therapy the pain and restriction can go on for many years. This wonderful and effective therapy can be a substitute for the drugs used in medicine that hide pain without healing it.

Structural balancing

As we age, there are many factors that can warp our posture. Gravity pulls down on us and some body parts seem to sag down. Work and play leave some parts stretched and other parts scrunched up. Special forms of massage have been developed to correct these postural changes. Ida Rolf did the groundbreaking research on the massage technique called "Rolfing".[8] This and many other structural alignment techniques can be used. Sitting in some chairs causes hunching and scrunching. Some work, especially deskwork, seems to cause the shoulders to hunch over. Underlying and surrounding our muscles there is a layer of dense myofascial tissue. This often looks like plastic wrap that has bunched up. There are well-known techniques for smoothing and moving this myofascial tissue. As the tissues are moved back into position, the posture relaxes. Vertebrae can float instead of being stacked like bricks. This relief is helpful in cases of herniated disks. The ribcage can float upward and the shoulders relax backward.

Muscle, tendon, and ligament injury

Most people experience muscle, tendon, or ligament injury many times in their lives. Massage therapies are the best way to heal and to prevent these injuries. This is often called "sports massage." Preventive massage therapy can find and relax tight tendons. Combined with stretching and warm-ups, massage can prevent many of these sports or work injuries. Shortened and tight ligaments can be identified and stretched by a good massage therapist.

As muscles are developed, they often get tight. This tightness and muscle stiffness leaves the muscles vulnerable to damage. Massage is excellent for finding and loosening these tight, new muscles. A tremendous amount of pain and lost work time is due to these problems. It is less effective to use drugs such as painkillers, anti-inflammatory drugs, and antispasmodics to hide the symptoms of these injuries after they occur.

Hydrotherapy

Hydrotherapy is the ancient and modern art of applying water at different temperatures to heal. We are all quite familiar with ice packs, but there is much more to the art of hydrotherapy. Ice packs are quite good at lessening the damage caused in the first few hours after a bruised or swollen injury. By keeping the swelling to a minimum, ice packs can reduce healing time. Ice packs can often be the wrong therapy or too strong of a therapy, however.

When there is a muscle spasm the ice pack can cause intensified spasms and ripped muscles. With muscle spasms, hot compresses, hot water bottles, and warm baths are recommended. Cold footbaths are great for relieving swollen, sore feet. Medicinal plants can be added to the water for astringent, antispasmodic, or relaxant effects.

Warm water can be applied in a variety of ways. Hot packs are excellent prior to massage of tight muscles. Hot packs are wet sand bags that are heated and placed on towels on the back and neck. Hot water bottles have been used throughout the ages to relax an area or aid in sleep. Hot water bottles are often used by women with menstrual cramps. Hot tubs can relax the whole person or water jets can be directed to relieve a sore muscle. Steam can be applied to the lungs or to the whole body. The addition of medicinal plants can also make these therapies much more effective.

Alternating hot and cold therapies noticeably speed up healing of injuries. The blood and toxins are squeezed out of the area by the cold water. The hot water allows fresh blood and nutrients to get into the relaxed capillaries again. Few people today have heard of *thalassotherapy*. This is a prescription to go swim in the ocean. The salt in the water pulls toxins through the skin while the trace minerals from the ocean water are absorbed. The relaxing effect is powerful.

Topical Applications

There are many topical applications that help make the various massage therapies more effective. Many massage therapies use oil for lubrication. This massage oil can have different essential oils added to it to get different effects. Some essential oils like blue chamomile oil (high in azulene) have a soothing, anti-inflammatory, and relaxing effect on injured tissue. Others like oil of wintergreen can have heating effects. These heating oils can pull the stagnant blood from underlying muscles into rapidly expanding surface capillaries. Often called balms, these skin-heating ointments can also rapidly relieve pain such as headache pain.

Ointments can soak into the body carrying nutrients to the underlying tissues. Some oils like castor oil have a special capacity for helping to reopen blocked lymph ducts. The smells of the various aromatherapy oils have a noticeable effect on the massage client. There are many other topical applications including poultices with herbs, fomentations (herb tea on a cloth), and clay packs. Modern medicine could improve patient care by learning more about these wonderful and effective techniques.

Teaching massage

One of the best ways a massage therapist can help people is to teach them to massage themselves and each other. Self-massage has the tremendous advantage in that you are able to feel the exact pressure needed. Once a person has experienced professional massage he can then work on himself to duplicate the massage. There are, however, areas and techniques that cannot be done by self-massage. That is why it is a great idea to have a relative or a friend attend the massage sessions to learn how to help with the specific therapies needed. Most of the massage techniques can be taught to an amateur in minutes. The person on the table can give feedback to the amateur therapist to adjust pressure or location. Because massage is often needed for repetitive stresses and injuries, these healing techniques can be used over and over.

HOMEOPATHIC REMEDIES

Homeopathic remedies are used throughout Europe, Great Britain, India, and much of the world. First of all, they do no harm. Their effects have been proven in multitudes of studies including double-blind studies.[9] The full-strength *mother tincture* is diluted and shaken many times to create the homeopathic remedy. Minerals, herbs, parts of animals, and other substances are used. Because of the dilution, homeopathic remedies have limited side effects in any normal dose. Many homeopathic remedies are sold over the counter in stores in America. Some, such as arnica, are widely used with obvious success. Medical science has a hard time understanding homeopathic remedies.

The theory of homeopathy depends on the two-step action of drugs. Step one is what the drug does to the body. Step two is how the body adapts. This adaptation is usually the opposite of the drug's action. Let us take as an example a person with a poison ivy rash. This person might be counseled to take some homeopathic *rhus tox*, which is made from diluted and shaken poison ivy tincture. This homeopathic remedy pushes the body just a little bit to increase the swelling and itching. Because of the extreme dilution, the symptoms are not actually worsened, or they are worsened only briefly. The body then pushes back harder to reduce the swelling. The net result is decreased swelling, itching, and burning.

One aspect of homeopathic prescribing for chronic disease is the incredibly detailed history of the person and their symptoms. Experts using books, personal experience, and/or computer programs are able to identify the correct remedy and dosage. While chronic disease prescribing in homeopathic medicine requires a long education, acute prescribing for first aid is easily learned in a few seminars. Doctors could learn how to use the most common homeopathic remedies. With low cost and low chance for harm, homeopathic medicine can be a wonderful alternative to dangerous drugs.

These and many other natural therapies need to be included in order for medicine to become complete. Open-minded doctors are learning about a new world of safer and gentler therapies.

Chapter 14

Food Supplements and Superfoods

To build toward optimum health we may find that we need some concentrated nutrient sources. There are many natural food supplements and superfoods that we can use to build our health wealth. These differ from chemical medicine in that they exist naturally in our food or are found naturally in our bodies. Many of these natural food supplements act on the whole body rather than on a particular organ or system. Many have antioxidant properties that help us maintain excellent health well into old age. These supplements tend to restore a natural balance in our bodies rather than having the overpowering effect that some drugs have. Instead of suppressing symptoms, they help our bodies to cure themselves. Doctors and their patients will find that restoring internal balance provides an enduring cure. These natural substances support health and keep us strong. The following supplements are some of the best.

Food Supplements

Acidophilus, the Friendly Bacteria

Acidophilus and other friendly bacteria (sometimes called *probiotics*) are important for smooth digestion. Antibiotics, coffee, oral contraceptives, corticosteroids, and alcohol reduce the amount of these necessary bacteria or mutate them into damaging forms.[1] Candida, gas, bloating, and constipation occur when the amount of friendly bacteria drops. Our bodies should have about eighty percent friendly lactobacillus acidophilus bacteria and twenty percent of the less friendly bacteria. The reverse is often true.[2] We need this bacterial balance to absorb vitamin B12. Vitamin B12 is vital for energy production. Vitamin B1,[3] vitamin B6,[4] and vitamin B2[5] can also be made in our intestines by friendly bacteria. These friendly acidophilus bacteria produce their own antibiotics to keep unfriendly bacteria and yeast at bay. These are the good germs.

Bioflavonoids

Bioflavonoids are part of the vitamin C complex. Our bodies need bioflavonoids and cannot make them. Their chief function is to strengthen our arterial walls, especially the walls of capillaries. Cardiovascular doctors can use bioflavonoid supplementation for protection from weak spots and ballooning in arterial walls (aneurysms). Bioflavonoids are needed to prevent and help cure bruises, varicose veins, hemorrhoids, strokes, and other circulatory disorders.[6] They are used for athletic injuries and cataracts as well. When taking vitamin C, bioflavonoids need to be taken along with the vitamin C to offset the slight tendency of vitamin C to encourage bleeding. Bioflavonoids are made from the white part of citrus fruits. Other sources include hesperidin, rutin, procyanidins, and quercitin. Bioflavonoids are sometimes referred to as vitamin P.

Bitters

Bitters are digestive aids made from various bitter medicinal plants such as gentian (*gentiana lutea*), rhubarb root (*rheum palmatum*), and dandelion root. They act upon the liver and gall bladder to release gall bile. These bitters are helpful with jaundice, gall bladder pain, hepatitis, and in the reduction of cholesterol. They can also be taken after a meal high in fats to relieve the sensation of fullness.

Most Americans get far too much in the way of sweets in their diet and beverages. The only bitter tastes usually found in American diets are coffee and a few bitter spices. Bitters offset the excess sugars and tighten and tone the whole system.

Bromelain

Bromelain is an enzyme derived from pineapples. It is used before and after sports injuries to protect and heal bruising and sprains. It acts as an anti-inflammatory and works well with bioflavonoids.[7] Bromelain is also a digestive enzyme. Sports injury specialists should know about bromelain.

Coenzyme Q10

Coenzyme Q10 is a powerful antioxidant. It is found throughout human tissue and is also known as *ubiquinone.* It reduces the side effects of chemotherapy and reduces deaths from tumors and leukemia.[8] It is used by the immune system and retards the aging process. Cardiologists should consider it for high blood pressure and arterial disease.[9] Allergy experts should consider it for allergies and asthma. Oncologists should realize its potential for controlling cancer. Psychiatrists should know that it can be used to treat schizophrenia and Alzheimer's disease. It is also used to treat multiple sclerosis and diabetes. One favorite use of Coenzyme Q10 is to stop or reverse periodontal disease, making gum surgery unnecessary in some cases. Because Coenzyme Q10 is gradually reduced in tissues as we age, it is wise to supplement it.

DHEA

Dehydroepiandrosterone (DHEA) is an adrenal hormone that declines as we age. It is the raw material from which we make male and female hormones. DHEA is synthesized from wild yam root. It is used to enhance energy and well-being. There is evidence that it is useful for lupus, for the immune system, and for osteoporosis.[10] It may be taken as a natural supplement. However, a better way is to enhance our body's own production of DHEA with exercise, relaxation techniques, outdoor time, a natural diet, and by limiting alcohol and caffeine intake.

Dimethylglycine

Vitamin B15 in the form of dimethylglycine (DMG) is

often taken for oxygen starvation. It helps in seconds when dissolved under the tongue. Vitamin B15 in the form of dimethylglycine helps transport oxygen into our cells for energy production and improves immune response.[11] It also decreases muscle fatigue by decreasing lactic acid in the blood.

Some years ago the Russians did a study on what factors in food are lost on the way to market. They discovered that vitamin B15 was one important lost nutrient. They discovered two forms of B15: pangamic acid and its calcium salt, dimethylglycine. Dimethylglycine is the active part of pangamic acid. Apparently, there was some industrial espionage that stole the wrong formula. The stolen formula was for pangamic acid. Although not as useful as DMG, some companies still sell pangamic acid.

Dimethylglycine is packaged in foil blisters for rapid absorption under the tongue. Athletes use it for high altitude and aerobically challenging exercise. People with angina, asthma, and emphysema also find relief from improved oxygen transport. It is found in whole grains, nutritional yeast, barley sprouts, and garden fresh green vegetables.

DLPA

The amino acid DL-Phenylalanine (DLPA) is effective for chronic pain, especially chronic back pain.[11] It is unique among painkillers in that it makes the mind more alert, not less alert. It has also been used to relieve depression. Because this amino acid is a component of protein, it is safe except in the rare condition of *phenylketonuria* (inability to tolerate the amino acid phenylalanine). Although DLPA may need some weeks to take effect, it is perfect for chronic pain. There are some people for whom DLPA has no effect. Therapists who treat back pain and other chronic pain could consider this natural alternative to chemical painkillers.

Garlic

Garlic is a powerful natural antibiotic. It kills some bacteria on contact. We should treat infectious diseases with
garlic and other natural antibiotics in preference to chemical antibiotics whenever possible. We can include garlic as a
part of the therapy for hypertension and arteriosclerosis.
Garlic is also very effective against worms in the digestive
tract. For those who don't enjoy the flavor of garlic in their
food, there are tablets and capsules of garlic that have been
deodorized. Garlic is best taken cooked or raw with other
food.

Ginseng

All of the types of ginseng revitalize the body. There are
three main types of ginseng, each with its own special properties. Panax Ginseng is the ancient Chinese root that is given
when frail old age starts to wither a person. It is also grown
in Korea. This ginseng is a powerful warming stimulant that
enriches, rather than depletes the strength. It stimulates the
hormone systems to revitalize strength and sexual potency.
This is a powerful root that must be used with care in
younger persons as it can create excessive energy and heat.

A second type of ginseng is Siberian Ginseng
(*eleutherococcus senticosus*). It is used for strength, stamina,
and endurance. Siberian ginseng does not increase heat in
the body; in fact it has been used to lessen the effects of heat
extremes. Siberian ginseng is popular among women who
wish to reduce hot flashes but maintain strength, athletes
who wish to burn energy smoothly, and people who generally wish to increase stamina without increasing heat in their

bodies. Siberian ginseng also has antioxidant properties.

A third type of ginseng is American Ginseng (*panax quinquefolium*). This root is a general tonic with special effects on skin and digestion. It is grown in North America and is highly prized by the Japanese and Chinese for its strong, clear properties of vigor and strength. All of these Ginseng roots require fifteen years of growing time before being considered prime quality.

Glucosamine Sulfate

Glucosamine sulfate and the somewhat similar chondroitin sulfate are both used for pain and arthritis. Glucosamine sulfate stimulates the repair of joint cartilage by supplying the raw materials needed. Chondroitin sulfate inhibits enzymes that destroy cartilage molecules. Chondroitin sulfate also facilitates maintaining the water cushions in cartilage; these water cushions are shock protecting and promote flexibility.[13]

Many doctors who treat arthritis know about these natural products. With the use of glucosamine sulfate and chondroitin sulfate, the progression of arthritis is slowed and the symptoms lessened. With seventy million Americans suffering from arthritis pain, relief is sorely needed from this painful and disabling disease.

Lecithin

Lecithin is found in every cell in the body. It is needed by, and in fact is a large component of, the cell membranes. Lecithin prevents hardening of the cell membranes so that nutrients can continue to pass through them. Lecithin prevents oxidation damage to cell walls and arteries. It also protects muscles, nerves, and our brains from oxidation damage. Lecithin is an emulsifier that allows fats like cholesterol to be dispersed in water and removed from our bodies.

Lecithin is composed of choline and inositol (B-vitamins), and the essential fatty acid linoleic acid. It is found in soybeans, whole grains, beans, wheat germ, and nutritional yeast. Although lecithin is also found in eggs, the accompanying cholesterol is excessive. Lecithin is important in preventing and treating hardening of the arteries, high cholesterol, high serum triglycerides, alcoholic liver damage, and elderly brain dysfunction.[14] Lecithin is a food component without harmful side effects when used in moderate amounts.

Lysine

The essential amino acid lysine is found in most normal foods. Amino acids are components of protein. When lysine is taken alone it stops herpes from growing in the body. Lysine supplementation is a harmless and powerful aid for these painful herpes sores. Chocolate, coffee, and foods high in the amino acid arginine encourage the growth of herpes. Arginine is found abundantly in nuts. In order to have a positive balance between lysine and arginine, nuts need to be reduced or offset by more lysine. Many people use lysine for prevention and treatment of ulcerated mouth sores. Lysine can often be used instead of painkillers for these conditions.

Octacosanol

Octacosanol is an energy factor found in the germ of wheat. Athletes have used it for years to enhance performance, especially endurance. It helps oxygen utilization in the cells and is used by high-altitude athletes and asthma sufferers. By helping our muscles store glycogen, octacosanol improves our stamina. Policosanol is composed primarily of octacosanol. Policosanol has been found to lower blood cholesterol by about twenty percent in human and animal tests.[15]

Propolis

Propolis is a substance collected by bees for use as glue and to protect their hive from bacteria and fungi. It is a very thick black goo. A diluted mixture of propolis and echinacea tincture is perfect for spraying into a sore throat. When used in a throat spray it is very effective in killing germs, soothing inflammation, and coating the throat. This mixture helps mucous membranes while activating the immune system.

Propolis can also be used in a salve to prevent infection with open wounds. Propolis is too sticky to use alone. It needs to be added to other things like throat spray or cough drops to become usable. It stimulates cytokine secretions that activate the immune system.[16]

Pycnogenol

Pycnogenol has powerful antioxidant properties, which makes it effective for a wide variety of problems caused by free radical damage. It works with vitamin C as a bioflavonoid to strengthen capillary walls and improve the elasticity of red blood cells. Pycnogenol also has an anti-inflammatory action. It is used for diabetic retinopathy, protection from ultraviolet skin damage, asthma, lupus erythematosus, premenstrual tension, and attention deficit disorder.[17]

The active ingredient in Pycnogenol is called *proanthocyanidin*, which is derived from Maritime Pine bark or from grapefruit seeds. This is the same substance that gives the red pigment to cabbage and it may play a role in

Some Great Natural Supplements

To Enhance Your Health

Acidophilus
Bioflavonoids
Bitters
Bromelain
Coenzyme Q10
DLPA
Garlic
Ginseng
Glucosamine sulfate
Chondroitin sulfate
Lecithin
Lysine
Octacosanol
Propolis
Pycnogenol
SOD
Trace minerals
Vitamin B15

the anti-ulcer properties of cabbage. Pycnogenol is used with bilberry for diabetic retinopathy.

Sam-e

Sam-e (S-adenosyl-l-methionine) is one of the best remedies for arthritis and other joint pain. It repairs damage to joints and helps to protect us from diseases of the brain and nervous system. Many important neurotransmitters like dopamine, norepinephrine, adrenaline, and serotonin need methylation—which Sam-e promotes. Methyl donors like Sam-e have also been shown to protect against gene damage that leads to cancer.

Sam-e acts as an antioxidant to protect us from damage to blood vessels. One way that Sam-e works is to promote our body's main antioxidant, glutathione. Sam-e also reduces the production of a toxic amino acid called homocysteine. This prevents homocysteine from damaging our arteries.[18]

Superoxide Dismutase

Superoxide Dismutase, often called *SOD*, is a powerful antioxidant. It is an enzyme that destroys *superoxide*, the most common of the free radicals in our bodies.[19] Healthy young bodies produce plenty of this anti-aging factor. With advancing age and poor health, less SOD is produced in our bodies. An enzyme called catalase works with SOD to reduce the rate of cell destruction from free radical action. A good superoxide dismutase supplement can contain five million units and be enteric coated. SOD is found in most green vegetables and especially in sprouts.

Trace Minerals

Trace mineral supplements give us all of the trace minerals that may be lacking in our food. Zinc, chromium, and molybdenum are some of the better-known trace minerals. We need only a little of them, but we still need them very much.[20] It is impossible to list all of the disease states that benefit from the use of trace minerals. It would be hard to find diseases that would not benefit.

Most of the agricultural soil in America is depleted of

many trace minerals. Trace mineral supplements are often made from ancient sea deposits or made from seaweed. Eating seaweed is one good way to get trace minerals, as long as the seaweed is harvested from a clean sea. When taken as a supplement, the trace minerals need to be taken in a balanced supplement such as chelated colloidal minerals.

SUPERFOODS

Superfoods are foods with concentrated nutrients. There is no clear delineation between supplements, medicinal plants, and superfoods. Superfoods are more food-like than most medicinal plants or supplements. They provide a nutritional impact that spirals health upwards. Superfoods often boost energy. In this age of chronic fatigue, we should be aware of concentrated food energy boosters. Some of the best superfoods are listed below.

Barley Greens

Barley greens are made by sprouting the grain of barley. Barley is one of the most ancient of cultivated grains. The grain is sprouted and planted in a tray of soil. The grass is harvested and juiced. The juice, fresh or reconstituted from dried barley sprouts, is a potent energizer. The analysis of barley grass has revealed that it is exceedingly high in many important vitamins and minerals. Barley grass contains an alkaloid, *gordenine*, which has an action similar to ephedrine.[21] This is why barley grass is used to relieve bronchitis. Dried barley grass mixed in water or juice is a refreshing beverage.

As a food, the barley grain is known for its strengthening and soothing properties. Cooked barley is also easy to digest and assimilate and has long been recommended for people recovering from illness.

Some Great Superfoods

Barley Greens
Bee Pollen
Chlorella
Spirulina
Flax Seed Oil
Gomasio
Kelp
Nutritional Yeast
Root Vegetables
Royal Jelly
Sprouts
Wheat Germ

Bee Pollen

Bee pollen is pollen that bees collect from flowers. It is an energizer. It is used by athletes to boost energy and endurance. It contains many needed nutrients such as calcium, complete protein, copper, DNA, RNA, enzymes, vitamins, twenty-seven mineral salts, iron, lecithin, magnesium, and zinc.[22] Sometimes screens are used in the entrance of beehives to collect the flower pollen.

The pollen should be from unsprayed flowers. It is best if the pollen is fresh or cracked to improve the availability of nutrients. Some pollen is quite delicious and satisfying to eat. Occasionally people with hay fever use a tiny amount of bee pollen before hay fever season begins, gradually building up their bee pollen dose to increase their resistance to airborne pollen. For this use it is best to get local pollen from a beekeeper. The person must build up the dosage slowly, to ensure that there is no bad reaction.

Chlorella

Chlorella is a single-celled algae farmed in ponds specially constructed for this purpose. A few grams provide a definite energy boost. Chlorella is a perfect supplement for those who cannot get enough fresh green food. The whole cell is used but is first subjected to a process in which the cell wall is fractured to improve digestibility. It is high in chlorophyll, which is nearly identical to hemoglobin. The available chlorophyll helps our bodies to make hemoglobin, thus enriching our blood. The extra hemoglobin transports more oxygen, which boosts energy. It is excellent for those with anemia. Chlorella contains about 60% protein with a complete complement of amino acids. Spirulina is a very similar superfood.

Flaxseed Oil

Flaxseed oil is pressed out of flax seed. It is the best source of essential fatty acids of the few foods that contain both of the essential fatty acids. These essential fatty acids are extremely hard to get in an American diet. The essential fatty acids help with any nervous system disorder, especially epilepsy, multiple sclerosis, and Alzheimer's disease.[23] The seeds of Flax are laxative, soothing, and anti-inflammatory.

Whole flax seeds have been used for the treatment of respiratory and digestive inflammatory disorders. It is interesting to note how they are used for this. The raw seeds are soaked overnight in a glass of water. The next morning, the water is consumed but the seeds are left in the glass. More water is added and the process is repeated for over a week, at which point the water becomes thick and milky and very soothing.

Ground flax seeds are also used externally as a poultice to relieve pain and heal skin wounds. The cooked oil is known as linseed oil. Linseed oil is no longer edible, but rather is used as a base for oil paints.

Gomasio

Gomasio is simply sesame seeds that have been lightly roasted with salt. The seeds are usually ground up after cooking. Gomasio is a delicious topping for many foods. Gomasio is a great way to get sesame seeds into the diet. Whole brown sesame seeds are the highest source of dietary calcium, even more concentrated than milk. Gomasio is used instead of salt to supply many nutrients including vitamin T.[24]

Kelp

Kelp is one of the many types of seaweed that are eaten. It is rich in trace minerals that are hard to get in an American diet. It is a salty food, so other sources of salt should be reduced when it is eaten. Kelp is often eaten in soups and stews. It can also be crumbled and sprinkled on top of food. It is a good source of easily assimilated iodine. Nori is another good seaweed. It is made into dried, flat sheets and wrapped around rice in Japanese food.

Nutritional Yeast

Nutritional yeast is loaded with vitamins and other needed nutrients. It is the highest source of dietary B-vitamins and has a noticeable effect as an energy booster. This may be partially due to the easily assimilable vitamin B12. Originally, brewer's yeast was used as the supplement. Now we have nutritional yeast, which is better tasting, fortified, and grown specifically for nutrients.

Nutritional yeast is high in a special form of chromium, which is very easy to assimilate.[25] This form of chromium is helpful with hypoglycemic problems such as mood swings because of the *Glucose Tolerance Factor*. Nutritional yeast has complete protein—about forty percent by weight. It needs to be added to rice, cereals, soups, or vegetables just prior to eating so that the fragile B-vitamins are not destroyed by cooking. It is quite popular as a flavoring for popcorn along with sea salt and vegetable seasoning.

Root Vegetables

Root vegetables include potatoes, carrots, beets, taro, yams, and sweet potatoes. These foods are deeply strengthening and stabilizing for the human body. To get the complete goodness from root vegetables, they should be cooked in soups, stews, or baked. These vegetables are hearty, solid foods that help with nervousness or weakness. They are helpful in recharging the depleted energy that characterizes so many Americans.

Royal Jelly

Royal jelly is the thick, milky substance secreted from the pharangeal glands of a special group of young nurse bees between their sixth and twelfth days of life. When royal jelly is fed to ordinary bees they become queen bees. It is often combined with honey to preserve its potency. It spoils easily so keep it refrigerated and tightly sealed. Royal jelly has antibacterial and antibiotic properties due to its ecanoic acid content.[26] In addition to containing all the major vitamins, it has enzymes and hormones. It is often taken to boost energy, enhance fertility, and promote healing.

Sprouts

Sprouts are foods that help us to be healthy and energetic. Many seeds can be sprouted. Some of the best sprouts are made from alfalfa seeds, mung beans, radish seeds, and red clover seeds. When seeds are germinated, many of their nutrients are made available. Sprouts are high in superoxide dismutase (SOD), which keeps us young and helps us to resist free radical damage.

Wheat Germ

Wheat Germ is the heart of the wheat kernel. Wheat germ oil is also used as a superfood and must be refrigerated and away from light. Wheat germ contains octacosanol, which is a powerful energy factor. Octacosanol helps our cells get oxygen. Wheat germ is also high in natural vitamin E, which is hard to get in our diet. In most commercial bread products, vitamin E has been removed, along with the entire wheat germ. When choosing bread products, try to find real whole wheat breads to enhance your health.

AFTERWORD

We have a long way to go to heal modern medicine. This healing can only be done by combining the best from natural medicine and the best from modern medicine. I hope this book will help doctors and patients understand how natural healing works. My goal is to outline what is missing from modern medicine so that it can be included. We need the current type of medical practice for emergencies and acute needs, supplemented with natural medicine. We need holistic practitioners for preventing and treating chronic disease, supplemented with modern medicine. Natural medicine is also the right choice for many other health problems that are not critical. Ideally, the two types of healing can be merged into one unified system.

Basic healthy lifestyles and habits are essential to prevent the current epidemics of chronic diseases. With pressure from millions of patients and also HMOs, doctors are looking at these natural ways of preventing disease. It is going to take a revolution in thinking for modern doctors to move away from using primarily drugs and surgery. New training courses need to be available for doctors who wish to learn these gentler and more effective ways to practice medicine. Pioneer doctors are practicing natural medicine right now and the patients are lining up.

Selected Bibliography:

Abehsera, Michel. *The Healing Clay*. Brooklyn, NY: Swan House, 1979.

Airola, Paavo. *How To Get Well*. Phoenix, AZ: Health Plus, 1974.

Anders, George. *Health Against Wealth*. New York: Houghton Mifflin, 1996.

Anthony, Catherine P., and Gary A. Thibodeau. *Textbook of Anatomy and Physiology*. St. Louis: Mosby, 1979.

Ashford, Nicholas A., and Claudia S. Miller. *Chemical Exposures*. New York: Van Nostrand Reinhold, 1991.

Ballentine, Rudolf. *Diet and Nutrition*. Honesdale, PA: Himalayan International Institute, 1978.

Beers, Mark H., and Robert Berkow. *The Merck Manual. 17th Edition*. Whitehouse Station, NJ: Merck, 1999.

Bieler, Henry G. *Food is Your Best Medicine*. New York: Vintage, 1973.

Black, Dean. *Health at the Crossroads*. Springville, UT: Tapestry Press, 1988.

Blake, Steve. *Natural Healing Solutions CD*. Haiku, HI: LifeLong Press, 2004.

Brown, Barbara B. *Stress and the Art of Biofeedback*. New York: Bantam, 1981. An excellent technical book about many biofeedback procedures.

Cameron, Ewan, and Linus Pauling. *Cancer and Vitamin C*. Menlo Park, CA: Linus Pauling Institute of Science and Medicine, 1979. An excellent book outlining decades of experience using ascorbated vitamin C with cancer patients. This book imparts a clear understanding of malignant diseases and their treatment.

Christopher, John R. *School of Natural Healing*. Provo, UT: BiWorld, 1976.

Clouatre, Dallas. *Glucosamine Sulfate and Chondroitin Sulfate*. Los Angeles: Keats, 1999.

Coulter, Harris L. *Divided Legacy: Science and Ethics in American Medicine*. Richmond, CA: North Atlantic Books, 1982.

Davis, Elizabeth. *A Guide to Midwifery, Heart and Hands.* Santa Fe, NM: John Muir Publications, 1981.

Epstein, Samuel S. *The Politics of Cancer.* San Francisco: Sierra Club Books, 1978. This whole book is an excellent expose of how politics corrupts science.

Erasmus, Udo. *Fats and Oils.* Burnaby, BC, Canada: Alive Books, 1986. This is an excellent book on dietary oils.

Feingold, B. F. *Why Your Child Is Hyperactive.* New York: Random House, 1985. A good reference for child reactions to food dyes, food additives, and food allergies.

Gofman, J. W. *Preventing Breast Cancer.* San Francisco: Committee for Nuclear Responsibility, Inc., 1996.

Gofman, J. W. and E. O'Conner. *X-Rays: Health Effects of Common Exams.* San Francisco: Sierra Club Books, 1985.

Hall, R. H. *Food for Naught: the Decline in Nutrition.* New York: Vintage Books, 1976. This is a classic book by a Canadian biochemistry professor.

Howells, William. *Mankind in the Making.* Garden City, NY: Doubleday, 1967.

Illich, Ivan. *Medical Nemesis.* New York: Pantheon Books, 1976.

Inlander, C., L. S. Levine, and E. Weiner. *Medicine on Trial.* New York: Pantheon Books, 1988.

Jensen, Bernard. *Nature Has A Remedy.* Santa Cruz, CA: Unity Press, 1978.

Jensen, Bernard, and Mark Anderson. *Empty Harvest.* Garden City Park, NY: Avery, 1990.

Johanson, David. *Lucy, the Beginnings of Mankind.* New York: Simon and Schuster, 1981.

Lander, L. *Defective Medicine.* New York: Farrar, Straus, Giroux, 1978.

Laws, Edward A. *Aquatic Pollution.* New York: John Wiley and Sons, Inc., 1993. This is a very comprehensive and scary book on water pollution. Professor Laws is the Chairperson of the Department of Oceanography at the University of Hawaii at Manoa.

Lesser, M. *Nutrition and Vitamin Therapy.* New York: Bantam, 1981.

Lewis, Walter H. *Medical Botany*. New York: John Wiley and Sons, 1977.

McArdle, William D., Frank Katch, and Victor Katch. *Exercise Physiology*. Philadelphia: Lea and Febiger, 1986.

Mendelsohn, R. S. *Confessions of a Medical Heretic*. Chicago: Contemporary Books, 1979.

Murray, Michael, and Joseph Pizzorno. *Encyclopedia of Natural Medicine*. Rocklin, CA: Prima, 1991.

Passwater, Richard A. *Supernutrition*. New York: Pocket Books, 1975.

Pauling, Linus. *Vitamin C, the Common Cold, and the Flu*. San Francisco: Freeman, 1976.

Pelletier, Kenneth R. *Mind as Healer, Mind as Slayer*. New York: Delta, 1977.

Pfeiffer, Carl C. *Mental and Elemental Nutrients*. New Canaan, CT: Keats, 1975.

Pfeiffer, Carl C. *Zinc and other Micronutrients*. New Canaan, CT: Pivot, 1978.

Preston, T. *The Clay Pedestal*. Seattle, WA: Madrona, 1981.

Regenstein, Lewis. *America the Poisoned*. Washington, DC: Acropolis Books, 1982. Read the introduction, and you will have no further doubts that America is poisoned.

Robbins, John. *Diet for a New America*. Walpole, NH: Stillpoint, 1987.

Robertson, W. O. *Medical Malpractice: A Preventive Approach*. Seattle: University of Washington Press, 1985.

Rolf, Ida P. *Rolfing: The Integration of Human Structures*. New York: Harper and Row, 1977. This book is a must for any body worker or anyone who strives to understand human structure.

Selye, H. *Stress Without Distress*. New York: Signet, 1994.

Sherman, Janette. *Chemical Exposure and Disease*. New York: Van Nostrand Reinhold, 1988. An excellent book for understanding occupational disease.

Smith, Jeffery. *Seeds of Deception*. Fairfield, IA: Yes! Books, 2003.

Stitt, Paul A. *Fighting the Food Giants*. Manitowoc, WI: Natural Press, 1981.

Waldbott, George L. *Health Effects of Environmental Pollutants*. St. Louis:

Mosby, 1973.

Weiss, Rudolf F. *Herbal Medicine*. Bath, Great Britain: The Bath Press, 1988. This is one of the best books on herbal medicine. Doctor Weiss is a medical doctor and also a leader in *phytotherapy* (plant medicine). His knowledge of medicinal plants is vast.

Weitz, M. *Health Shock*. Englewood Cliffs, NJ: Prentice-Hall, 1982.

West, John B., Ed. *Best and Taylor's Physiological Basis of Medical Practice*. Eleventh Edition. Baltimore, MD: Williams and Wilkins, 1985.

Williams, Roger J. *Biochemical Individuality*. New York: Wiley, 1979. This excellent book details the differences between the structure and biochemistry of different people. Actual autopsy drawings show how different our organs are from one person to another.

Williams, Roger J. *Nutrition Against Disease*. New York: Pitman, 1980.

Winter, Ruth. *A Consumer's Dictionary of Food Additives*. New York: Crown Publishers, 1978. This is an excellent reference.

Winter, Ruth. *A Consumer's Dictionary of Household, Yard, and Office Chemicals*. New York: Crown Publisher's, Inc., 1992.

Zamm, Alfred V. *Why Your House May Endanger Your Health*. New York: Touchstone, 1980.

Chapter 1

1. A. Castiglioni, *A History of Medicine* (New York: Alfred A. Knopf, 1958), p. 172.

2. Harris L. Coulter, *Divided Legacy, Science and Ethics in American Medicine* (Richmond, CA: North Atlantic Books, 1982). The whole book discusses this division.

3. *Best and Taylor's Physiological Basis of Medical Practice*, Eleventh Edition, Ed., John B. West (Baltimore, MD: Williams and Wilkins, 1985), p. 892. This reference addresses the suppression of hormones after hormone replacement therapy.

4. R. Clement, "Resistant Germs, Resistant Physicians," *BioMedical Therapy* 15:3 (June 1997): 68.

5. Rudolf Ballentine, *Diet and Nutrition* (Honesdale, PA: Himalayan International Institute, 1978), p. 76.

6. *Physiological Basis of Medical Practice*, Ed., John B. West, 892.

7. Rosemary Gladstar, *Herbal Healing for Women* (Rockefeller Center, NY: Fireside, 1993), p. 148.

8. Linus Pauling, *Vitamin C, the Common Cold, and the Flu* (San Francisco: Freeman, 1976), p. 67.

9. Ballentine, *Diet and Nutrition*, 99, 100, 102.

10. G. Canguilhem, *Le Normal et la Pathalogique* (Paris: Presses Universitaires de France, 1972). Good Health was not always understood as simply freedom from clinical signs.

11. Bernard Jensen and Mark Anderson, *Empty Harvest* (Garden City Park, NY: Avery, 1990), p. 40.

12. Alfred V. Zamm, *Why Your House May Endanger Your Health* (New York: Touchstone, 1980), p. 24. This book is a good introduction to indoor air and the pollutants that it contains.

13. Janette Sherman, *Chemical Exposure and Disease* (New York: Van Nostrand Reinhold, 1988), pp. 58-59.

14. Henry G. Bieler, *Food is Your Best Medicine* (New York: Vintage, 1973), p. 193.

Chapter 2

1. Roger J. Williams, *Biochemical Individuality* (New York: Wiley, 1979).

2. R. M. Poses, et al., "The Accuracy of Experienced Physicians' Probability Estimates for Patients with Sore Throats," *Journal of the American Medical Association* 254:7 (August 16, 1985): 927.

3. B. C. Coleman, "MDs Flunk Test to Find Cancerous Breast Lumps," (New Brunswick, N.J) *The Home News*, 19 April 1985, sec. A, p. 6.

4. S. Epstein, R. Bertell, and B. Seaman, "Dangers and Unreliability of Mammography: Breast Examination is a Safe, Effective, and Practical Alternative," *International Journal of Health Services*, 31:3 (2001): 605-615. Also See S. Weed, Menopausal Years, the Wise Woman Way (Woodstock, NY: Ashtree, 1992), p. 102.

5. Weed, *Menopausal Years*, 102.

6. John William Gofman, *Preventing Breast Cancer* (San Francisco: Committee for Nuclear Responsibility, Inc., 1996).

7. Bernard Jensen and Mark Anderson, *Empty Harvest* (Garden City Park, NY: Avery, 1990), p. 116.

8. "Mammography not Fail-Safe, Doctors Caution," (New Brunswick, NJ) *The Home News*, 24 January 1986, sec. A, p. 6.

9. E. K. Koranyi, "Morbidity and Rate of Undiagnosed Physical Illnesses in a Psychiatric Clinic Population," *Archives of General Psychiatry* 36 (April 1979): 414-416. Also see A. Smith, "Primary Care MDs Overlook 90% of Psychiatric Illnesses," *Clinical Psychiatry News* 12:2 (February 1984): 1, 27.

10. George Anders, *Health Against Wealth* (New York: Houghton Mifflin, 1996), p. 133.

11. N. Brozan, "Doctors Learning to Diagnose Alcoholism," *New York Times*, 16 December 1985, p. 16.

12. *U.S. Department of Health and Human Services, Centers for Disease Control and Prevention, National Center for Health Statistics*, "Advance Data From Vital and Health Statistics," No. 321 (November 1, 2001).

13. Anders, *Health Against Wealth*, 8.

14. Ibid., 76.

15. *Health and Human Services*, "Advance Data."

Chapter 3

1. J. J. Brokaw, G. Tunnicliff, B.U. Raess, and D.W. Saxon, "The Teaching of Complementary and Alternative Medicine in U.S. Medical Schools: A Survey of Course Directors," *Academic Medicine: Journal of the Association of American Medical Colleges* 77:9 (September 2002): 876-881.

2. P. D. Clote, "Automated Multiphasic Health Testing: An Evaluation," *Antologia A* (1974): 8.

3. John R. Christopher, *School of Natural Healing* (Provo, UT: BiWorld, 1979), pp. 359-360.

4. L. J. Mata, et al., "Host Resistance to Infection," *American Journal of Clinical Nutrition* 24 (August 1971): 976-986.

5. U. Heininger, J. D. Cherry, et al., "Comparative Efficacy of the Lederle/Takeda Acellular Pertussis Component DPT (DTaP) Vaccine...in German Children After Household Exposure," *Pediatrics* 102:3 (September 1998): 546.

6. J. B. Robbins, R. Schneerson, and B. Trollfors, "Pertussis in Developed Countries," *Lancet* 360:9334 (August 31, 2002): 657.

7. A. J. Wakefield, et al., "Ileal-lymphoid-nodular hyperplasia, nonspecific colitis, and pervasive developmental disorder in children," *Lancet* 351: 9103 (February 28, 1998): 637.

8. C. M. Benjamin, G. C. Chew, and A. J. Silman, "Joint and Limb Symptoms in Children After Immunization with Measles, Mumps, and Rubella Vaccine," *British Medical Journal* 304:6834 (April 25, 1992): 1075. This study shows a six times increase in pain and swelling in children's joints within six weeks of immunization.

Chapter 4

1. American Heart Association, *2002 Heart and Stroke Statistical Update* (Dallas, Texas: American Heart Association, 2001).

2. *American Heart Association, for the year 1999*. (American Heart Association, Inc. [cited 6 July, 2002]); available from http// :www.americanheart.com; INTERNET.

3. *American Heart Association, for the year 1999*. INTERNET. This figure includes lost work productivity.

4. George Anders, *Health Against Wealth* (New York: Houghton Mifflin, 1996), p. 96.

5. Ibid., 106.

6. K. A. Bauman, "The Family Physician's Reasonable Approach to Upper Respiratory Tract Infection Care for this Century," *Archives of Family Medicine* 9:7 (July 2000): 596-597.

7. A. Aubertin, "Not All Bacteria Are Bad: Probiotics Promise Help to G.I. Tract, Immunity," *Environmental Nutrition* 24:11 (November 2001): 1-2.

8. K. Rankin, "New Treatment Options Help Battle a Killer: Prostate Disorders," *Drug Store News* 19:11 (July 14, 1997): CP7.

9. Ibid.

10. C. B. Inlander, *This Won't Hurt* (Allentown, PA: People's Medical Society, 1998), p. 120.

11. Michel Abehsera, *The Healing Clay* (Brooklyn, NY: Swan House, 1979), p. 8.

12. Steve Blake, *Alternative Remedies (St. Louis: Mosby, 1979).*

Chapter 5

1. Kenneth R. Pelletier, *Mind as Healer, Mind as Slayer* (New York: Delta, 1977), p. 40.

2. C. Kohn, S. Hast, and C. W. Henderson, "Chronic Stress can Interfere with Normal Function of the Immune System," *Immunotherapy Weekly* (December 4, 2002): 2.

3. Barbara B. Brown, *Stress and the Art of Biofeedback* (New York: Bantam, 1981), pp. 155-160. An excellent book about many biofeedback procedures.

4. Steve Blake, tests with the Trifield meter in magnetic field detection mode in a number of cars has led me to this conclusion.

5. Pelletier, *Mind as Healer*, 168.

6. R. Martin, *The Gravity Guiding System* (Pasadena, CA: Gravity Guidance, Inc., 1981) A good introduction to inversion by the inventor of excellent inversion equipment.

7. M. Walker and F. Angelo, *Rebounding Aerobics* (Edmonds, WA: The National Institute for Reboundology and Health, Inc., 1981), p. viii.

8. Pelletier, *Mind as Healer*, 134. This is a reference to family stress causing cancer. This excellent book shows links to many other diseases.

9. B. F. Feingold, *Why Your Child Is Hyperactive* (New York: Random House, 1985). A good reference for child reactions to food dyes, food additives, and food allergies.

10. R. H. Hall, *Food for Naught: the Decline in Nutrition* (New York: Vintage Books, 1976). This classic book by a Canadian biochemistry professor outlines these contaminants.

11. Alfred V. Zamm, *Why Your House May Endanger Your Health* (New York: Touchstone, 1980), pp. 78-79.

12. Edward A. Laws, *Aquatic Pollution* (New York: John Wiley and Sons, Inc., 1993). This is a very comprehensive and scary book on water pollution. Professor Laws was the Chairperson of the Department of Oceanography at the University of Hawaii at Manoa. This book is an authoritative overview of water pollution.

13. Ronald R. Parks, (Asheville, NC [cited 19 September, 2002]); available from http//:www. macrohealthmedicine.com; INTERNET).

14. Brown, *The Art of Biofeedback*, 155-160.

15. H. Selye, *Stress Without Distress* (New York: Signet, 1994), p. 74. An excellent book on stress and its effect on us.

16. Pelletier, *Mind as Healer*. Starting on page 229, this book will introduce you to Autogenic Relaxation and other forms of relaxation.

Chapter 6

1. Bernard Jensen and Mark Anderson, *Empty Harvest* (Garden City Park, NY: Avery, 1990), p. 148.

2. Roger J. Williams, *Biochemical Individuality* (New York: Wiley, 1979). This excellent book details the differences between the

structure and biochemistry of different people. Actual autopsy drawings show how different our organs are from one person to another.

3. Florence Lin, *Chinese Vegetarian Cookbook* (Boulder, CO: Shambala, 1983). This is an excellent book for finding substitutes for meat. One secret of the Orient is using wheat gluten as a meat substitute.

4. Nicholas A. Ashford and Claudia S. Miller, *Chemical Exposures* (New York: Van Nostrand Reinhold, 1991), p. 35. This is a technical book on Clinical Ecology, the study of addiction and allergy to substances.

5. Rudolf Ballentine, *Diet and Nutrition* (Honesdale, PA: Himalayan International Institute, 1978), pp. 433-441.

6. R. G. Windsor, "Nutritional Education for Doctors Lacking," *Spectrum: The Wholistic News Magazine* 18 (May/June 1991): 13.

7. R. H. Hall, *Food for Naught: the Decline in Nutrition* (New York: Vintage Books, 1976), p. 47.

8. David Johanson, *Lucy, the Beginnings of Mankind* (New York: Simon and Schuster, 1981), pp. 320-321 (hands) and p. 267 (teeth).

9. Ballentine, *Diet and Nutrition*, 117.

10. Johanson, Lucy, *The Beginnings of Mankind*, 286-287.

11. William Howells, *Mankind in the Making* (Garden City, NY: Doubleday, 1967), p. 205. We have only been making sharp stone tools for about thirty-five thousand years. Without these flint tools, butchery was difficult.

12. "Stopping the Madness," *Satya, a Magazine of Vegetarianism, Environmentalism, and Animal Advocacy* (January, 1988).

13. Johanson, *Lucy, The Beginnings of Mankind*, 40. There is a quote on this page from an earlier anthropologist, Raymond Dart, where humans are, "…slaking their ravenous thirst with the hot blood of victims and greedily devouring livid, writhing flesh."

14. Howells, *Mankind in the Making*, 173.

15. Ibid., 145.

16. M. B. Snell, "Gorillas in the Crossfire," *Sierra* 86:6 (November/December 2001): 30.

17. P. A. Apoil, F. Roubinet, S. Despiau, et al., "Evolution of alpha 2-fucosyltransferase genes in primates: relation between an intronic Alu-Y element and red cell expression of ABH antigens," *Molecular biology and Evolution* 17:3 (March 2000): 337-351.

18. R. Z. Hawkins, "Seeing Ourselves as Primates," *Ethics & the Environment* 7:2 (Autumn 2002): 60.

19. Johanson, *Lucy, The Beginnings of Mankind*, 270.

20. Howells, *Mankind in the Making*, 92.

21. Ibid., 120.

22. D. C. Johanson, "Human Origins," *National Forum* 76:1 (Winter 1996): 24.

23. J. H. Tilden, *Toxemia Explained* (New Canaan, CT: Keats, 1981), p. 92.

24. Linus Pauling, *Vitamin C, the Common Cold, and the Flu* (San Francisco: Freeman, 1976), pp. 76-77.

25. N. Altman, *Eating for Life: the Ultimate Diet* (NY: Vegetus Books, 1984). Also see: *Facts of Vegetarianism*, (Dodgeville, NY: North American Vegetarian Society, 1970), P. 5.

26. C. Lo, "Integrating Nutrition as a Theme Throughout the Medical School Curriculum," *American Journal of Clinical Nutrition* 72:3 Supplement (September 2000): 882S-889S.

27. Steve Blake, *Nutrient Wizards CD-ROM* (Honopou, HI: LifeLong Press, 2004), www.naturalhealthwizards.com.

28. William D. McArdle, Frank Katch, and Victor Katch, *Exercise Physiology* (Philadelphia: Lea and Febiger, 1986), p. 86.

29. Ibid., 80.

30. Catherine P. Anthony and Gary A. Thibodeau, *Textbook of Anatomy and Physiology* (St. Louis: Mosby, 1979), p. 509.

31. McArdle, *Exercise Physiology*, 96.

32. Paul A. Stitt, *Fighting the Food Giants* (Manitowoc, WI: Natural Press, 1981). This is a good book on nutrient depletion in foods written by a biochemist who worked for a leading food company.

33. Ballentine, *Diet and Nutrition*, 520. Dr. Ballentine outlines the burning of extra vitamin C here. The B-vitamins are also depleted with stress. For depletion of nutrients with pollution, see George L. Waldbott, *Health Effects of Environmental Pollutants* (St. Louis: Mosby, 1973), p. 91.

34. Lewis Regenstein, *America the Poisoned* (Washington, DC: Acropolis Books, 1982), p. 82.

35. Edward A. Laws, *Aquatic Pollution* (New York: John Wiley and Sons, Inc., 1993), p. 277. This page has a chart showing water levels of DDT (an organochlorine pesticide) at 0.00005 parts per million. As the food chain is followed and bigger fish eat smaller fish, and birds eat fish, the levels rise to 26.4 parts per million.

36. Regenstein, *America the Poisoned*, 15-18. Read the introduction on these pages and you will have no further doubt that America is poisoned.

37. Laws, *Aquatic Pollution*, 258.

38. George L. Waldbott, *Health Effects of Environmental Pollutants* (St. Louis: Mosby, 1973), p. 222.

39. Hall, *Food for Naught*, 109-114.

40. S. Epstein, "The Chemical Jungle: Today's Beef Industry," *International Journal of Health Services* 20:2 (1990): 277-280.

41. S. Globus, "Pros and Cons of Food Additives," *Current Health* 2 28:2 (October 2001): 17. Also see: Institute of Food Technologists, "Nitrites, Nitrates, and Nitrosamines in food—a dilemma," *Food Technology* 26:11 (1972): 121-124.

42. K. W. Rubin, "Benefits and Pitfalls: Antioxidants and Health," *Foodservice Director* 14:9 (September 15, 2001): 64. Also see: S. S. Mirvish, et al., "Ascorbate-Nitrite Reaction: Possible Means of Blocking the Formation of Carcinogenic N-Nitroso Compounds," *Science* 177 (1972): 65-67.

43. Beatrice Trim Hunter, *Beatrice Trim Hunter's Additives Book* (New Canaan, CT: Keats, 1980), p. 105.

44. *Best and Taylor's Physiological Basis of Medical Practice, Eleventh Edition*, Ed., John B. West (Baltimore, MD: Williams and Wilkins, 1985), p. 506.

45. Jeffery Smith, *Seeds of Deception*, (Fairfield, IA: Yes! Books, 2003), p. 95-96.

46. McArdle, *Exercise Physiology*, 545.

47. John Robbins, *Diet for a New America* (Walpole, NH: Stillpoint, 1987), p. 292.

48. E. Ward, "Many Protective Nutrients Needed to Keep Bones Healthy and Fracture-Free," *Environmental Nutrition* 22:12 (December 1999): 1. Also see: F. Ellis, et al., "Incidence of Osteoporosis in Vegetarians and Omnivores," *American Journal of Clinical Nutrition* 25 (1972): 555-558.

49. Jensen, *Empty Harvest*, 47.

50. Carl C. Pfeiffer, *Mental and Elemental Nutrients* (New Canaan, CT: Keats, 1975), pp. 23-24.

51. *U.S. Department of Health, Education, and Welfare*, "Report of the Secretary's Commission on Pesticides and Their Relationship to Environmental Health, Parts 1 and 2," (Washington, DC: U.S. Department of Health, Education, and Welfare, 1969).

52. D. Pimentel and H. Acquay, "Environmental and Economic Costs of Pesticide Use," *Bioscience* 42:10 (November 1992): 750.

53. Regenstein, *America the Poisoned*, 103-104.

54. Wataru Takahashi, *Pesticide Usage Patterns in Hawaii, 1977* (Honolulu, HI: Pacific Biomedical Research Center, May 24, 1982), p. 48.

55. Marc Lappé and Britt Bailey, *Against the Grain: Biotechnology and the Corporate Takeover of Your Food*, (Monroe, ME: Common Courage Press, 1998), p. 76.

56. Smith, *Seeds of Deception*, 39. This book documents many cases of interference with safety testing by the genetically modified food and drug industries.

57. Stitt, *Fighting the Food Giants*, 143-146.

58. Ruth Winter, *A Consumer's Dictionary of Household, Yard, and Office Chemicals* (New York: Crown Publisher's, Inc., 1992), p. 92. Chlorine dioxide is a highly irritating and corrosive gas.

59. K. L. Fortmann, et al., *Wheat Pigments and Flour Color, Wheat Chemistry and Technology*, Edited by Y. Pomerantz (St. Paul, MN: American Association of Cereal Chemists, 1971), pp. 493-522.

60. Laws, *Aquatic Pollution*, 249.

61. Hall, *Food for Naught*, 22. A classic book on how food is ruined by technology.

62. S. H. Webster, et al., "The Toxicology of Potassium and Sodium Iodates. III. Acute and Subacute Oral Toxicity of Potassium Iodate in Dogs," *Toxicology Applied Pharmacology* 8 (1966): 185-192.

63. Hall, *Food for Naught*, 27.

64. Code of Federal Regulations, Title 21, Volume 2, Revised as of April 1, 2002, From the *U.S. Government Printing Office* via GPO Access (CITE: 21CFR101.4).

65. Anthony, *Textbook of Anatomy and Physiology*, 515.

66. U.S. Department of Agriculture, Agricultural Research Service, USDA Nutrient Data Laboratory, *USDA Nutrient Database for Standard Reference, Release 14* (July, 2001).

67. Ibid.

68. Hall, *Food for Naught*, 247.

69. Winter, *Household, Yard, and Office Chemicals*, 47.

70. Ibid., 193-194.

71. Hall, *Food for Naught*, 243-245.

72. Waldbott, *Health Effects of Environmental Pollutants*, 56. Many other pages offer explanations of how these toxins affect health.

73. Winter, *Household, Yard, and Office Chemicals*, 265, 268, 50.

74. R. Keuneke, "Health Destructive Effects of Frying," *Total Health* 21:3 (July/August 1999): 26.

75. Hall, *Food for Naught*, 243-245.

76. J. Gorman, "Trans Fats," *Science News* 160:19 (November 10, 2001): 300.

77. Janette Sherman, *Chemical Exposure and Disease* (New York: Van Nostrand Reinhold, 1988), p. 108.

78. Kim Severson, "Trans Fat in Food: As Bad As It Gets," *San Francisco Chronicle*, 11 July, 2002, sec. A, pp. 1, 5, 6.

79. Kim Severson, "Hidden Killer, It's Trans Fat. It's Dangerous. And It's In Food You Eat Every Day," *San Francisco Chronicle*, 30 January 2002.

80. J. Gorman, "Trans Fats," *Science News* 160:19 (November 10, 2001): 300.

81. Severson, "Trans Fat in Food," sec. A, 1, 5, 6.

82. Severson, "Hidden Killer, It's Trans Fat."

83. W. C. Willett, M. J. Stampfer, et al., "Intake of Trans Fatty Acids and Risk of Coronary Heart Disease among Women," *The Lancet* 341:8845 (March 6, 1993): 581-585.

84. *A Physician's Handbook on Orthomolecular Medicine*, Eds., Roger J. Williams, et al. (New Canaan, CT: Keats, 1977), p. 125.

85. The American Heart Association reports in 2002 that there are sixty million Americans with some form of heart disease and 1.1 million heart attacks yearly. (*American Heart Association, Inc.* [cited 6 July, 2002]); available from http//:www.americanheart.com; INTERNET.

Chapter 7

1. D. T. DeVita, "A Perspective on the War on Cancer," *Cancer Journal* 8:5 (September/October 2002): 352-357.

2. L. Tomatis, "Etiologic Evidence and Primary Prevention of Cancer," *Drug Metabolism Reviews* 32:2 (May 2000): 129. A great article with actual lists of human carcinogens. For the increase in cancer cases and deaths see: S. Epstein, "Reversing the Cancer Epidemic," *Tikkun* 17:3 (May 2002): 56. He shows a 58% increase in cancer cases in the last half of the last century of which only a quarter are smoking-related.

3. George Anders, *Health Against Wealth* (New York: Houghton Mifflin, 1996, p. 116.

4. Ewan Cameron and Linus Pauling, *Cancer and Vitamin C* (Menlo Park, CA: Linus Pauling Institute of Science and Medicine, 1979). An excellent book outlining decades of experience using ascorbated vitamin C with cancer patients. This book imparts a clear

understanding of the different malignant diseases and how they can be treated.

5. Coogan, et al., "Exposure to Power Frequencies," *Archives of Environmental Health* 53:5 (1998): 359.

6. Alfred V. Zamm, *Why Your House May Endanger Your Health* (New York: Touchstone, 1980), p. 81.

7. Isobel Smith, "Electromagnetic Radiation and Health Risks: Cell Phones and Radiation in New Zealand," *Journal of Environmental Health* 59:1 (July-August, 1996): 19.

8. D. Leszczynski, S. Joenväärä, J. Reivinen, and R. Kuokka, "Non-Thermal Activation of the Hsp27/P38mapk Stress Pathway by Mobile Phone Radiation in Human Endothelial Cells: Molecular Mechanism for Cancer and Blood-Brain Barrier-Related Effects," *Differentiation* 70:2/3 (May 2002): 120.

9. B. F. Feingold, *Why Your Child Is Hyperactive* (New York: Random House, 1985), p. 161. A good reference for child reactions to food dyes, food additives, and food allergies.

10. Feingold, *Why Your Child Is Hyperactive*, 123.

11. S. Epstein, "Reversing the Cancer Epidemic," *Tikkun* 17:3 (May 2002): 56.

12. Feingold, *Why Your Child Is Hyperactive*, 123.

13. L. Berry, "Internal Cleansing," *Alive: Canadian Journal of Health and Nutrition* 185 (March 1998): 60.

14. Ruth Winter, *A Consumer's Dictionary of Food Additives* (New York: Crown Publishers, 1978). This is an excellent reference. She also has a guide for household and yard chemicals.

15. Lewis Regenstein, *America the Poisoned* (Washington, DC: Acropolis Books, 1982), p. 189.

16. John R. Christopher, *School of Natural Healing* (Provo, UT: BiWorld, 1976), pp. 518-519. Dr. Christopher was a pioneer in developing the "mucusless diet."

17. Janette Sherman, *Chemical Exposure and Disease* (New York: Van Nostrand Reinhold, 1988), pp. 61, 67.

18. Ibid.

19. Zamm, *Why Your House*, 114-116. There is a nice table of non-toxic alternative pest control on these pages

20. Mark H. Beers and Robert Berkow, *The Merck Manual, 14th Edition* (Whitehouse Station, NJ: Merck, 1982). Strangely enough, the bad news about this drug has been removed from newer editions of this manual.

21. Michael Culbert, *Medical Armageddon* (San Diego, CA: C and C Communications, 1997).

22. Edward A. Laws, *Aquatic Pollution* (New York: John Wiley and Sons, Inc., 1993), p. 165.

23. Ibid., 175-176.

24. C. Prater and R. G. Zylstra, "Autism: A Medical Primer," *American Family Physician* 66:9 (November 1, 2002): 1667.

25. Ellen Moyer, *Minerals* (Allentown, PA: People's Medical Society, 1997), p. 149-200.

26. California Environmental Protection Agency, Department of Pesticide Regulation, *Sampling for Pesticide Residues in California Well Water, 2002 Update of the Well Inventory Database*, EH02-07 (December 2002) p. ii.

Chapter 8

1. *A Physician's Handbook on Orthomolecular Medicine*, Eds., Roger J. Williams, et al. (New Canaan, CT: Keats, 1977), p. 1.

2. D. McGuire and M. Morris, "Bold Moves are Needed to Protect Public from Dangerous Pharmacies, Experts Say," (Kansas City, MO) *The Kansas City Star*, 8 October 2002.

3. FDA Drug Review; "Postapproval Risks 1976-85", *United States General Accounting Office* (GAO) GAO/PEMD-90-15, April 1990. The severe postapproval risks considered were adverse reactions that could lead to hospitalization, increases in the length of hospitalization, severe or permanent disability, or death.

4. Ivan Illich, *Medical Nemesis* (New York: Pantheon Books, 1976), p. 74.

5. K. A. Galt, "Medication Errors in Ambulatory Care," *Topics in Health Information Management* 23:2 (November 2002): 36. Also see:

J. Brown, D. Stephen, F. Landry, "Recognizing, Reporting, and Reducing Adverse Drug Reactions," *Southern Medical Journal* 94:4 (April, 2001). Also see: J. Lazarou, B. Pomeranz, and P. Corey, "Incidence of adverse drug reactions in hospitalized patients: a meta-analysis of prospective studies," *Journal of the American Medical Association* 279:15 (April 15, 1998).

6. Galt, "Medication Errors in Ambulatory Care," 34.

7. C. B. Inlander, *This Won't Hurt* (Allentown, PA: People's Medical Society, 1998), p. 123.

8. Galt, "Medication Errors in Ambulatory Care," 35.

9. E. B. Larson, "Inadequate Medical Order Writing: A Source of Confusion and Increased Costs," *Western Journal of Medicine* 139:1 (July, 1983): 50.

10. C. Inlander, e.t al., *Medicine on Trial* (New York: Pantheon Books, 1988), p. 147.

11. P. H. Peristein, et al., "Errors in Drug Computations During Newborn Intensive Care," *American Journal of Diseases of Childhood* 133 (April 1979): 376.

12. *Parents Guide to Prevention: Growing Up Drug-Free* (Pueblo, CO: National Clearing House for Drug Information 1993). D. R. Lamb, "Anabolic Steroids in Athletics: How Well Do They Work and How Dangerous Are They?" *American Journal of Sports Medicine* (January-February 1984): 31-38.

13. Illich, *Medical Nemesis*, 26.

14. B. Starfield, "Is the U.S. Health Really the Best in the World?" *Journal of the American Medical Association* 284:4 (July 26, 2000).

15. C. W. Stratton, "Pulmonary Infections in Critical Care Medicine—the Wright State University School of Medicine Symposium: Bacterial Pneumonias—an Overview with Emphasis on Pathogenesis, Diagnosis and Treatment," *Heart and Lung* 15:3 (May 1986): 226-244.

16. K. L. Melmon, "Preventable Drug Reactions—Causes and Cures," *New England Journal of Medicine* 284:24 (June 17, 1971): 1361.

17. C. W. Burt, "Trends: National Trends In Use Of Medications In Office-Based Practice, 1985-1999," (*Centers for Disease Control's National Center for Health Statistics*, 2002).

18. W. O. Robertson, *Medical Malpractice: A Preventive Approach* (Seattle: University of Washington Press, 1985), p. 77.

19. Ibid., 187.

20. M. Weitz, *Health Shock* (Englewood Cliffs, NJ: Prentice-Hall, 1982), p. v.

21. R. Sullivan, "Number of Doctors Selling Prescription Drugs Grows," *New York Times*, 19 March 1987, sec. B, pp. 1, 5.

22. Weitz, *Health Shock*, v.

23. L. Lander, *Defective Medicine* (New York: Farrar, Straus, Giroux, 1978), p. 45.

24. J. A. Johnson and J. L. Bootman, "Drug-Related Morbidity and Mortality," *Archives of Internal Medicine* 55:18 (October 9, 1995): 1949. Also see: K. Steel, et al., "Iatrogenic Illness on a General Medical Service at a University Hospital," *New England Journal of Medicine* 304 (March 12, 1981): 638-642.

25. Starfield, "Is the U.S. Health Best."

26. Mark H. Beers and Robert Berkow, *The Merck Manual, 17th Edition*, (Whitehouse Station, NJ: Merck, 1999), pp. 1637-1643.

27. "Diazepam Tablets," *Clinical Pharmacology* (January 1, 2001).

28. T. Pugh, "Drug Reps Get the Cold Shoulder," *Toronto Star* 6 September 2002.

29. T. Zoellner, "America's Other Drug Problem," *Men's Health* 16:8 (October 2001): 118.

30. National Center For Policy Analysis, "Up to 5 Percent of Clinical Trials May Be Fraudulent," *Daily Policy Digest, Health Issues / Drug Research & Development*, Friday, February 08, 2002.

31. Chan, An-Wen, et al., "Empirical Evidence for Selective Reporting of Outcomes in Randomized Trials: Comparison of Protocols to Published Articles," *Journal of the American Medical Association* 291:20 (May 2004):2457-2465.

32. U.S. Senate, Select Committee on Small Business, Subcommittee on Monopoly, *Competitive Problems in the Drug*

Industry, 90th Congress, 1st and 2nd Sessions, 1967-1968, pt. 2, p. 565.

33. Ibid.

34. J. F. Hellegars, "Chloramphenicol in Japan: Let it Bleed," *Bulletin of Concerned Asian Scholars* 5 (July 1973): 37-45.

35. G. J. Povar, et al., "Patients' Therapeutic Preferences in an Ambulatory Care Setting," *American Journal of Public Health* 74:12 (December 1984): 1395-1397.

36. Dean Black, *Health at the Crossroads* (Springville, UT: Tapestry Press, 1988), p. 66.

37. S. Epstein, "Reversing the Cancer Epidemic," *Tikkun* 17:3 (May 2002): 56.

38. Victor J. Schoenbach, ([cited September 9, 2002]); available from http//:www.www.epidemiolog.net; INTERNET.

39. C. B. Inlander and E. Weiner, *Take This Book to the Hospital with You* (Emmaus, PA: Rodale Press, 1986), pp. 121-122.

40. *Hospital Infections*, Eds., A. E. Buxton, J. V. Bennett, and P. S. Brachman (Philadelphia, PA: Lipencott-Raven Publishers, 1998), p. 99.

41. S. B. Levy, "The Challenge of Antibiotic Resistance," *Scientific American* 278:3 (March 1998): 46-54. Also see: American Iatrogenic Association Home Page, ([cited July 2002]); available from http//:www.iatrogenic.org; INTERNET.

42. S. B. Levy, "The Challenge of Antibiotic Resistance," *Scientific American* 278:3 (March 1998): 46-54. Also see: M. J. Blaser, " Infectious Diarrheas: Acute, Chronic and Iatrogenic," *Annals of Internal Medicine* 105:5 (November 1986): 786.

43. Lander, *Defective Medicine*, 49.

44. "Ties Yeast Infection Increase to Iatrogenic Causes," *Family Practice News* (July 1-14, 1983): 18.

45. N. Pfeiffer, "Newer Agent Steps in as Vancomycin Fails With Infections," *Dermatology Times* 21:12 (December 2000): 41.

46. Inlander, *This Won't Hurt*, 148.

47. R. L. Goforth and C. R. Goforth, "Appropriate Regualtion of Antibiotics in Livestock Feed," *Boston College Environmental Affairs Law Review* 28:1 (Fall 2000): 39-78.

48. American Iatrogenic Association Home Page.

49. A. Romano, M. J. Torres, et al., "Immediate Hypersensitivity to Cephalosporins," *Allergy* 57:6 (June 2002): 52.

50. U.S. Senate, *Problems in the Drug Industry*, pt. 2, 565.

51. Janette Sherman, *Chemical Exposure and Disease* (New York: Van Nostrand Reinhold, 1988), p. 64.

52. M. Rimpler, "Ginseng: Adaptogenicity, Part 2," *Biological Therapy* 14:4 (October 1996): 242. Also see: Walter H. Lewis, *Medical Botany* (New York: John Wiley and Sons, 1977), p. 373.

53. U. S. Food and Drug Administration (April 20, 2001[cited July, 2002]); Available from http://www.FDA.GOV/bbs/topics/ CONSUMER/CON00027.html; INTERNET.

54. S. Sellman, "What You Were Never Told About The Pill," *Healthy and Natural Journal* 7:32 (February 2000): 90.

55. Gina Kolata, "Hormone Replacement Study Abruptly Halted, Stunning Finding—Drugs Increase Breast Cancer Risk," *San Francisco Chronicle*, 9 July 2002, sec A, p. 3.

56. Steven Smith, "Estrogen Linked to Ovarian Cancer, Second Study's Results may Be Death Knell for Hormone Therapy," *San Francisco Chronicle*, 17 July 2002, sec. A, pp. 1, 6. This report is on a National Cancer Institute study.

57. Gina Kolata and Melody Peterson, "Hormone Replacement Study a Shock to the Medical System," *The New York Times*, 10 July 2002, sec. A, pp. 1, 16.

58. M. A. Block, "Overmedication of Hyperactive Children," (Washington, DC: Federal Document Clearing House, Inc., September 26, 2002) *House Government Reform Committee*.

Chapter 9

1. M. J. Berens, "Infection Epidemic Carves Deadly Path," *Chicago Tribune* (July 21, 2002). Also see S. W. Key, "Hospital Infections,

Drug Resistance Rise in U.S.," *Health Letter on the CDC* (March 23, 1998): 11.

2. S. W. Key, "Hospital Infections, Drug Resistance Rise in U.S.," *Health Letter on the CDC* (March 23, 1998): 11-12.

3. R. W. Dubois and R. H. Brook, "Preventable Deaths: Who, How Often, and Why?," *Annals of Internal Medicine* 109 (October 1, 1988): 586.

4. C. B. Inlander, "They Should Know Better," *People's Medical Society Newsletter* 18:2 (April, 1999): 3.

5. W. O. Robertson, *Medical Malpractice: A Preventive Approach* (Seattle: University of Washington Press, 1985), p. 77.

6. A. de la Sierra, et al., "Iatrogenic Illness in a Department of General Internal Medicine: A Prospective Study," *Mount Sinai Journal of Medicine* 56:4 (September, 1989): 267-271.

7. N. Baba and K. Shaar, "Nutritional Assessments of Patients and Adequacy of Diet in Selected Hospitals," *Journal of Nutritional Medicine* 4:3 (1994): 297-311.

8. Ibid., 297-311.

9. R. S. Mendelsohn, *Confessions of a Medical Heretic* (Chicago: Contemporary Books, 1979), p. 91.

10. P. A. Janssen, V. L. Holt and S. J. Myers, "Licensed, Midwife-Attended, Out-of-Hospital Births in Washington State: Are They Safe?," *Birth* 21:3 (September 1994): 141-148.

11. Elizabeth Davis, *A Guide to Midwifery, Heart and Hands* (Santa Fe, NM: John Muir Publications, 1981), p. vii.

12. R. Goodell and J. Gurin, "Where Should Babies Be Born?" *American Health* (January-February, 1984): 72. Also see: H. Goer, "The Assault on Normal Birth: The OB Disinformation Campaign," *Midwifery Today* 63 (Fall 2002): 10-15.

13. E. Kolbert, "Midwives Face Threat of High Insurance Cost," *New York Times*, 29 September 1985, p. 56.

14. C. Cancila, "Midwives Again Lose Liability Insurance Coverage," *American Medical News* (October 18, 1985): 16.

15. The Institute of Medicine, "Medical Professional Liability and the Delivery of Obstetrical Care: Volume I," *National Academy Press* (1989).

16. T. Ball and A. Wright, "Health Care Costs of Formula-Feeding in the First Year of Life," *Pediatrics* 103:4 part 2 (April 1999): 870-876.

17. D. Sudnow, *Passing On: The Social Organization of Dying* (Englewood Cliffs, NJ: Prentice-Hall, 1967).

18. C. Inlander, et al., *Medicine on Trial* (New York: Pantheon Books, 1988), p. 213.

Chapter 10

1. Thomas J. Moore, *Prescription for Disaster* (New York, Simon & Schuster, 1998). This book is filled with examples of dangerous prescription medications.

2. W. J. Hrushesky, "Circadian Timing of Cancer Chemotherapy," *Science* 228 (April, 1985): 73-75.

3. M. Dean, "Out of Step with the Lancet Homeopathy Meta-Analysis: More Objections than Objectivity?" *Journal of Alternative & Complementary Medicine* 4:4 (Winter 1998): 389.

4. Samuel S. Epstein, *The Politics of Cancer* (San Francisco: Sierra Club Books, 1978). This whole book is an excellent exposé of how politics corrupts science.

5. Eyal Press and Jennifer Washburn, "The Kept University," *The Atlantic Monthly*, 285:3 (March 2000): 39. An excellent article on conflict of interest and testing bias.

6. Ibid.

7. K. Schneider, "Faking It: The Case Against Industrial BioTest Laboratories," *Amicus Journal* 4 (Spring 1983): 14-25.

8. Tamar Nordenberg, "When Is A Medical Product Too Risky?" *FDA Consumer* 33:5 (September/October 1999): 8.

9. Moore, *Prescription for Disaster*, 167. There are many examples on this page of drugs with terrible side effects remaining on the market.

10. Howie Kurtz, "Research Labs Safety Tests Are Questioned," *The Washington Star*, July 1981, sec. A, p. 3. Also see: K. Schneider, "Faking It: The Case Against Industrial BioTest Laboratories," *Amicus Journal 4* (Spring 1983): 14-25.

11. Associated Press, "U.S. Charging 4 Falsified Reports on Drugs in Lab," *The New York Times*, 23 June 1981. Also see Howie Kurtz, "Research Labs Safety Tests Are Questioned," *The Washington Star*, July 1981, sec. A, p. 3.

12. Ian Gallagher, et al., "Mobile Phones Cover-Up," *The Express* (UK), Oct. 16, 1999.

13. A. J. Wakefield, et al., "Ileal-lymphoid-nodular hyperplasia, non-specific colitis, and pervasive developmental disorder in children," *Lancet* 351: 9103 (February 28, 1998): 637.

14. Air and Energy Engineering Research Laboratory, "Results of Sampling Program for Emissions from Sugarcane Field Burning— Hawaii, April 1986," (Washington, DC: *United States Environmental Protection Agency*, August, 1987), EPA-600/X-x87-240.

15. Epstein, *The Politics of Cancer*, 167.

16. Jeffery Smith, *Seeds of Deception*, (Fairfield, IA: Yes! Books, 2003), p. 111-123. This chapter documents the tryptophan disaster.

17. "The Doctors," *Nation* 260:2 (January 9, 1995): 56-60.

18. Ron Winkens, "Rational, cost effective use of investigations in clinical practice," *British Medical Journal* 324:7340 (March 30, 2002): 783.

19. Ibid.

20. Ibid. Also see: E. T. Wong, et al., "Ready! Fire!... Aim! An Inquiry into Laboratory Test Ordering," *Journal of the American Medical Association* 250:18 (November 11, 1983): 2511.

21. S. F. Kronlund and W. R. Phillips, "Physician Knowledge of Risks of Surgical and Invasive Diagnostic Procedures," *Western Journal of Medicine* 142:4 (April 1985): 565-569.

22. Ruth Winter, *A Consumer's Dictionary of Household, Yard, and Office Chemicals* (New York: Crown Publisher's, Inc., 1992), p. 65.

23. C. Inlander, et al., *Medicine on Trial* (New York: Pantheon Books, 1988), p. 45. Also see: T. Marshall and A. Rouse, "Blood

Pressure Measurement: Doctors Who Cannot Calibrate
Sphygmomanometers Should Stop Taking Blood Pressures," *British
Medical Journal* 322:7295 (October 6, 2001): 1167-1170.

24. D. K. Sur, et al., "Accuracy of electrocardiogram reading by
family practice residents," *Family Medicine* 32:5 (May 2000): 315-9.

25. John William Gofman, "Radiation From Medical Procedures in
the Pathogenesis of Cancer and Ischemic Heart Disease: Dose-
Response Studies With Physicians per 100,000 Population," (San
Francisco: *Committee for Nuclear Responsibility, Inc.*, 1999).

26. K. Wilson, "Storage Plays a Crucial Role in Handling
Computer-based Patient Medical Records," *Cisco World* (November
2001).

27. J. W. Gofman and E. O'Conner, *X-Rays: Health Effects of
Common Exams* (San Francisco: Sierra Club Books, 1985), p. 310.

28. A. L. Huebner, "X-rays, Cancer and Heart Disease," *World & I*
15:4 (April 2000): 168-174. Also see: M. Ko, "Radiation: Cure or
Cause?," *Report / Newsmagazine* (Alberta Edition) 28:2 (January 22,
2001): 46.

29. M. Weitz, *Health Shock* (Englewood Cliffs, NJ: Prentice-Hall,
1982), p. 89.

30. Gofman, *X-Rays: Health Effects*, 13.

31. Weitz, *Health Shock*, 89.

32. Gofman, *X-Rays: Health Effects*, 370.

33. E. P. Sonnex, A. D. Tasker, and R. A. Coulden, "The Role of
Preliminary Interpretation of Chest Radiographs by Radiographers in
the Management of Acute Medical Problems Within a Cardiothoracic
Centre," *British Journal of Radiology* 74:879 (March 2001): 230.

34. R. L. Dabice, "Pap Test Utility Compromised by Mistakes,"
Medical Tribune (September 4, 1985): 19.

35. Inlander, Medicine on Trial, 102.

36. E. Kuon, "Radiation dose reduction in invasive cardiology by
restriction to adequate instead of optimized picture quality," *Health
Physics* 84:5 (May 2003): 626-631. Also see: E. Manuel-Rimbau, et
al., "Iatrogenic vascular lesions after cardiac catheterization" *Revista
Espanola de Cardiologia* 51:9 (September 1998): 750.

37. "More lab mistakes in doctors' offices," *New York Times* (February 11, 1998): p. A16. Also see: Physician-Office Lab Results Less Accurate than Those of Licensed Labs, Study Shows," *Medical World News*, 25:7 (April 9, 1984):46.

38. Physician-Office Lab Results Less Accurate than Those of Licensed Labs, Study Shows," *Medical World News*, 25:7 (April 9, 1984): 47.

Chapter 11

1. C. B. Inlander, *This Won't Hurt* (Allentown, PA: People's Medical Society, 1998), p. 6.

2. T. G. Gutheil, et al., "Malpractice Prevention through the Sharing of Uncertainty," *New England Journal of Medicine* 311:1 (July 5, 1984): 50.

3. George Anders, *Health Against Wealth* (New York: Houghton Mifflin, 1996), pp. 85-86.

4. J. B. Hull, "Patients Are Often the Last People to See Their Own Medical Records," *Wall Street Journal*, 30 September 1985, pp. 2, 23.

5. J. F. Burnum, "La Maladie du Petit Papier: Is Writing a List of Symptoms a Sign of an Emotional Disorder?" *New England Journal of Medicine* (September 12, 1985): 690.

6. V. Guarner, "Unnecessary operations in the exercise of surgery. A topic of our times with serious implications in medical ethics," *Gaceta Medica de Mexico* 136:2 (March/April 2000): 183. Also see: C. Inlander, et al., *Medicine on Trial* (New York: Pantheon Books, 1988), p. 113.

7. *Cost and Quality of Health Care: Unnecessary Surgery: Report / by the Subcommittee on Oversight and Investigations of the Committee on Interstate and Foreign Commerce*, House of Representatives, Ninety-fourth Congress, second session. Washington, DC: U.S. Government Printing Office, 1976. v, 52 p. ; 24 cm. Call Number: RA410.53 .U52 1976; GovDoc: Y 4.In 8/4:H 34/25. It seems that no federal, general investigation of unnecessary surgeries has been done since this report.

8. "'Iatrogenic Disease' Now Third Biggest Killer in U.S.," *International Council for Health Freedom Newsletter* 4:4 (Winter 2000-2001): 47.

9. E. C. Pierce, Jr., "Anesthesiology," *Journal of the American Medical Association* 254:16 (October 25, 1985): 2318.

10. J. B. Cooper, et al., "Anesthesia Can Be Safer," *Medical Instrumentation* 19:3 (May-June 1985): 105.

11. Gennjoui, "Breaking the Oath: Are Some Doctors Performing Unnecessary Surgery?" *Hahnemann University* (Summer 1985): 11.

12. "House Report Says 23 Percent of Lens Implants Not Necessary," *Hospitals* (September 1, 1985): 52

13. A University of Michigan Health Minute Update on Important Health Issues, "Hysterectomy: It's not the only choice anymore, U-M doctors say New clinic focuses on alternative procedures for fibroids and bleeding," (Ann Arbor, MI: *University of Michigan Health Minute Update on Important Health Issues*, July, 2002).

14. C. Inlander, et al., *Medicine on Trial* (New York: Pantheon Books, 1988), p. 114.

15. Gordon Shields, "The Tonsils and Adenoids in Pediatric Patients," *Grand Rounds Presentation*, (Department of Otolaryngology, UTMB, June 19, 2002).

16. Inlander, *Medicine on Trial*, 114.

17. Inlander, *This Won't Hurt*, 14.

18. E. Eckholm, "Curbs Sought in Caesarean Deliveries," *New York Times*, 11 August 1986, sec. A, p. 10.

19. Inlander, *This Won't Hurt*, 14.

20. *The Public Citizen Health Research Group*, "It is estimated that half of the nearly one million cesarean sections done every year in the United States are medically unnecessary," (Washington, D.C. [cited 28 July, 2002]); available from http//:www.Childbirth.org; INTERNET.

21. R. S. Mendelsohn, *Confessions of a Medical Heretic* (Chicago: Contemporary Books, 1979), p. 54.

22. U. S. Veteran's Administration, Coronary Artery Bypass Surgery Cooperative Study Group, "Eleven-Year Survival in the Veteran's Administration: Randomized Trial of Coronary Bypass

Surgery for Stable Angina," *New England Journal of Medicine* 311:1 (1984): 1333-1339.

23. L. Lander, *Defective Medicine* (New York: Farrar, Straus, Giroux, 1978), pp. 54-55.

24. Inlander, *Medicine on Trial*, 159.

25. Inlander, *This Won't Hurt*, 105.

26. R. Sullivan, "Cuomo Proposes Periodic Reviews for All Doctors," *New York Times*, 29 May 1986, sec. B p. 8.

27. L. Shearer, "Intelligence Report: Ask the Doctor," *Parade* (October 3, 1982): 8.

28. R. J. Feinstein, "The Ethics of Professional Regulation," *New England Journal of Medicine* 312:12 (March 21, 1985): 803.

29. "A System Whose Ills Can Be Fatal," *Detroit Free Press*, 1 April 1984, sec. A, p. 1.

30. J. Brinkley, "Medical Discipline Laws: Confusion Reigns," *New York Times*, 3 September 1985, sec. B, p. 6.

31. C. R. Robinson, "Why the Conspiracy of Silence Won't Die," *Medical Economics* (February 20, 1984): 180.

32. F. Charatan, "Few Incompetent Doctors are Reported to US National Data Bank," *British Medical Journal* 322:7299 (June 9, 2001): 1383. Also see: H. H. Keyser, *Women Under the Knife* (Philadelphia: George F. Stickley, 1984), p. 6.

33. Ivan Illich, *Medical Nemesis* (New York: Pantheon Books, 1976), p. 85.

34. B. Starfield, "Is the U.S. Health Really the Best in the World?" *Journal of the American Medical Association* 284:4 (July 26, 2000).

35. M. J. Cetron and O. Davies, "Trends Now Changing the World," *Futurist* 35:1 (January/February 2001): 30-44. Also See: *Medical Geography: Techniques and Field Studies*, ed., N. D. McGlashan (New York: Barnes and Noble, 1973).

36. M. H. Liang, et al., "Chinese Health Care: Determinants of the System," *American Journal of Public Health* 63 (February 1973): 102-110.

37. Illich, *Medical Nemesis*, 15.

38. Ibid., 16.

39. S. Epstein, "Reversing the Cancer Epidemic," *Tikkun* 17:3 (May 2002): 56-66. For Breast cancer see: E. F. Lewison, "An Appraisal of Long-Term Results in Surgical Treatment of Breast Cancer," *Journal of the American Medical Association* 186 (1963): 975-978.

Chapter 12

1. R. G. Windsor, "Nutritional Education for Doctors Lacking," *Spectrum: The Wholistic News Magazine* 18 (May/June 1991): 13.

2. S. Davies, "Nutritional Flat-Earthers," *Journal of Nutritional Medicine* 1:3 (1990): 167. Also see: Linus Pauling, *Vitamin C, the Common Cold, and the Flu* (San Francisco, CA: Freeman, 1976), p. 189.

3. R. Cohen, S. Fallon, L. Horowitz, and B. Clement, "Vegetarianism vs. the Traditional Diet: Which is Better for Your Health?," *Consumer Health Newsletter* 24:4 (April 2001): 1-6. Also see: F. Ellis, et al., "Incidence of Osteoporosis in Vegetarians and Omnivores," *American Journal of Clinical Nutrition* 25 (1972): 555-558.

4. P. Bhaskaram, "Micronutrient Malnutrition, Infection, and Immunity: An Overview," *Nutrition Reviews* 60:5 (May 2002): S40-S46.

Chapter 13

1. Steve Blake, *Natural Healing Solutions* (Haiku, HI: LifeLong Press, 2004). All of these remedies can be found on this CD-ROM encyclopedic resource. Available from www.naturalhealthwizards.com.

2. Steve Blake, *Natural Healing Solutions.*

3. Rudolf F. Weiss, *Herbal Medicine* (Bath, Great Britain: The Bath Press, 1988). This is one of the best books on herbal medicine. Doctor Weiss was a medical doctor and also a leader in phytotherapy (plant medicine). His knowledge of medicinal plants is comprehensive and from many decades of experience.

4. Y. Sun, et al., "Immune Restoration and/or Augmentation of Local Graft Versus Host Reaction by Traditional Chinese Medicinal Herbs," *Cancer* 52 (July 1, 1983): 70-73.

5. Dean Black, *Health at the Crossroads* (Springville, UT: Tapestry Press, 1988), p. 114.

6. T. Scarman, "The Healing Properties of Rose Water and Rose Oil," *Positive Health* 73 (February 2002): 19-22.

7. Catherine P. Anthony and Gary A. Thibodeau, *Textbook of Anatomy and Physiology* (St. Louis: Mosby, 1979), p. 591.

8. Ida P. Rolf, *Rolfing: The Integration of Human Structures* (New York: Harper and Row, 1977). This book is a must for any body worker or anyone who strives to understand human structure.

9. K. Linde, N. Clausius, G. Ramirez, et al., "Are the Clinical Effects of Homeopathy Placebo Effects? A Meta-analysis of Placebo-Controlled Trials," *Lancet* 350:9081 (September 20, 1997): 834. Also see: M. Dean, "Out of Step with the Lancet Homeopathy Meta-Analysis: More Objections than Objectivity?" *The Journal of Alternative and Complementary Medicine* 4:4 (1998): 389.

Chapter 14

1. Bernard Jensen, *Nature Has A Remedy* (Santa Cruz, CA: Unity Press, 1978), p. 68.

2. Ibid.

3. V. Najar and E. Holt, "The Biosynthesis of Thiamin in Man," *Journal of the American Medical Association* 123 (1943): 683.

4. Rudolf Ballentine, *Diet and Nutrition* (Honesdale, PA: Himalayan International Institute, 1978), pp. 184-185.

5. V. Najar et al, "The Biosynthesis of Riboflavin in Man," *Journal of the American Medical Association* 126 (1944): 357-358.

6. L. Packer, G. Rimbach, and F. Virgili, "Antioxidant Activity and Biologic Activities of a Procyanidin-Rich Extract from Pine (Pinus Maritima) Bark, Pycnogenol," *Free Radical Biology and Medicine* 27:5-6 (September 1999): 704-724. Also see: Michael Lesser, *Nutrition and Vitamin Therapy* (New York: Bantam, 1981), pp. 84-85.

7. Michael Murray and Joseph Pizzorno, *Encyclopedia of Natural Medicine* (Rocklin, CA: Prima, 1991), p. 515.

8. F. Brugè, L. Tiano, T. Cacciamani, F. Principi, G. Littarru, "Effect of UV-C mediated oxidative stress in leukemia cell lines and its relation to ubiquinone content," *Biofactors* 18:1-4 (2003). Also see: S. Hodges, and N. Hertz "CoQ10: could it have a role in cancer management?" *Biofactors* 9:2-4 (1999).

9. S. T. Sinatra, "CoQ-10 for Anti-Aging and a Healthy Heart," *Total Health* 23:2 (March/April 2001): 42-44.

10. Beth M. Ley, *DHEA: Unlocking the Secrets to the Fountain of Youth* (Newport Beach, CA: BL Publications, 1996).

11. C. D. Graber, J. M. Goust, et al., "Immunomodulating Properties of Dimethylglycine in Humans," *Journal of Infectious Diseases* 143:1 (January 1981): 101-105. Also see: Richard A. Passwater, *Supernutrition* (New York: Pocket Books, 1975), p. 43.

12. Murray, *Encyclopedia of Natural Medicine*, 496.

13. Dallas Clouatre, *Glucosamine Sulfate and Chondroitin Sulfate* (Los Angeles: Keats, 1999).

14. Roger J. Williams, *Nutrition Against Disease* (New York: Pitman, 1980), p. 76.

15. I. Gouni-Berthold and H. K. Berthold, "Policosanol: Clinical Pharmacology and Therapeutic Significance of a New Lipid-Lowering Agent," *American Heart Journal* 143:2 (February 2002): 356-365.

16. C. Bratter, M. Tregel, C. Liebenthal, and H. D. Volk, "Prophylactic Effectiveness of Propolis for Immunostimulation: A Clinical Pilot Study," *Forsch Komplementarmed* 6:5 (October 1999): 256-260.

17. P. Rohdewald, "A Review of the French Maritime Pine Bark Extract (Pycnogenol), a Herbal Medication with a Diverse Clinical Pharmacology," *International Journal of Clinical Pharmacology and Therapeutics* 40:4 (April 2002): 158-168.

18. Dallas Clouatre, *All About SAM-e* (Garden City Park, NY: Avery, 1999).

19. D. W. Martin, P. A. Mayes, and V. W. Rodwell, *Harper's Review of Biochemistry*, 18th Edition (Los Altos, CA: Lange Medical Publications, 1981), p. 129.

20. Carl C. Pfeiffer, *Mental and Elemental Nutrients* (New Canaan, CT: Keats, 1975).

21. Steve Blake, *Natural Healing Solutions* (Haiku, HI: LifeLong Press, 2004).

22. H. F. Loomis, "The Perfect Food," *American Chiropractor* 23:2 (2001): 16-19.

23. Udo Erasmus, *Fats and Oils* (Burnaby, BC, Canada: Alive Books, 1986), pp. 260-266. There are many other pages with information on flax oil in this excellent book on oils.

24. Paavo Airola, How To Get Well (Phoenix, AZ: Health Plus, 1974), p. 273.

25. Pfeiffer, Mental and Elemental Nutrients, 290-293.

26. T. B. Orr, "Royal Jelly the Beehive: Fit for a Queen," Better Nutrition 60:7 (July 1998): 34.

Index

Please consider these other works by Steve Blake:

Herbal Property Dictionary by Steve Blake, AHG, MH. Over 900 properties are defined from well-known actions such as *stimulant,* to uncommon properties such as *alexeteric.* Medicinal plants from Western, Chinese, and Ayurvedic traditions, as well as essential oils, are covered. Thousands of examples of herbs with these properties are included. This is a comprehensive computer reference dictionary of herbal property definitions. 258 page PDF book. 2004. $18.95, LifeLong Press, www.NaturalHealthWizards.com (free sample available).

Medicinal Plant Names by Steve Blake, AHG, MH. Common names of herbs are easy to translate to botanical names with this essential guide. Quickly look up foreign names for medicinal plants in many languages—includes 7900 names from 35 countries. This is an indispensable guide to all who work with medicinal plants. 313 page PDF book. 2004. $18.95, LifeLong Press, www.NaturalHealthWizards.com (free sample available).

Medicinal Plant Actions by Steve Blake, AHG, MH. This essential reference guide lists actions and properties of over 700 medicinal plants. The number of agreeing references is included. This helps you to see which actions are attributed to a plant by multiple authors. For example, 13 authors agree that licorice is demulcent, while just one author lists licorice as antidepressant. 185 page PDF book. 2004. $12.95, LifeLong Press, www.NaturalHealthWizards.com (free sample available).

Constituents of Medicinal Plants by Steve Blake, AHG, MH. This definitive work presents over 3000 chemical constituents of medicinal plants. Definitions for about one third of these constituents are included. From Abetic acid to Zizyphic acid, herbalists will appreciate learning about these constituents and the plants that contain them. 914 pp. PDF book. 2004. $22.95, LifeLong Press, www.NaturalHealthWizards.com (free sample available).

Medicinal Plant Constituents by Steve Blake, AHG, MH. Have you ever wondered which chemical constituents were in ginger root? This herbal reference provides the answers for over 600 herbs. You will find exact information on the amount of minerals, vitamins, flavonoids, and thousands of other constituents in *Medicinal Plant Constituents*. 542 pp. PDF book. 2004. $18.95, LifeLong Press, www.NaturalHealthWizards.com (free sample available).

Natural Healing Solutions Software by Steve Blake, AHG, MH. Comprehensive and easy to find information. This is the master database for world knowledge of 1,377 natural medicines. Over 122,000 footnotes document accurate information from hundreds of books and journals from 35 countries. This advanced search engine allows multiple keywords. For example, you can find herbs that are sedative, helpful with jaundice, and have tannins. Software for Windows. 2004. $199.50, LifeLong Press, www.NaturalHealthWizards.com.

Aromatherapy and Essential Oils: A Complete Guide by Steve Blake, AHG, MH. Over one hundred essential oils are covered. You can quickly learn which oils have been used for hundreds of health conditions. Essential oil properties and constituents are arranged to show cross-cultural convergence. Usage notes and cautions are included along with ten thousand footnotes. Software for Windows. 2004. $69.95, LifeLong Press, www.NaturalHealthWizards.com.

Ayurvedic Remedies Software by Steve Blake, AHG, MH. This huge database of herbs and remedies from East Indian Ayurveda explores remedies, including herbs and formulas, from the Ayurvedic tradition. Comprehensive and easy to use information is included for 360 Ayurvedic remedies with over 60,000 footnotes. Software for Windows. 2004. $39.95, LifeLong Press, www.NaturalHealthWizards.com.

Chinese Patent Remedy Software by Steve Blake, AHG, MH. Quick and accurate information on the 68 most commonly used Chinese patent remedies. See where our favorite authors agree with over 4000 footnotes. Software for Windows. $49.95, LifeLong Press, www.NaturalHealthWizards.com.

Nutrient Wizards CD-ROM
by Steve Blake

Color charts display the nutrition in your daily diet.

See at a glance which foods are health building and which foods are depleting for your family. See your daily intake of vitamins, minerals, protein, fats and other nutrients.

- Colorful Charts display vitamins, minerals, calories and more.
- 67 Nutrients evaluated.
- 6000 foods are listed from the USDA's latest Food Composition Tables.
- The Wizard can teach you how to improve your food choices.
- Find out which foods are giving you the most vitamins.
- Protein quality is shown with colorful charts of amino acids.
- If one of your nutrients is low, foods high in that nutrient can be displayed.
- Eleven personalized categories for you - from young children to mature adults.

36 color charts included

LifeLong Press, www.NaturalHealthWizards.com.
Designed for Windows from Win 95 to Win XP

Natural Healing Solutions by Steve Blake

Comprehensive and easy to use software

This is the master database for world knowledge of 1,377 natural medicinals!

Includes: Medicinal plants, vitamins, minerals, nutritional supplements, formulas, essential oils, homeopathy, Ayurvedic remedies, foods, Chinese herbs & formulas.

- Colorful Plant Photos - Hundreds of them!
- Summaries of Herbs, Vitamins, and Minerals.
- 32,200 Health Condition listings.
- Dosage and Warning information.
- Need Stimulant or Sedative information? 19,800 Action listings are available!
- Find the ingredients of your favorite formulas.
- Help is on every page and sensitive to your needs.
- Explore Herbal Constituents — 28,500 listings.
- Definitions will help you to understand new words.
- Find alternate herb names from around the World — over 11,000 listings.

Over 122,000 footnotes document accurate information from hundreds of books and journals from 35 Countries.

www.naturalhealthwizards.com
Designed for Windows from Win 95 to Win XP

Aromatherapy and Essential Oils

A Complete Guide by Steve Blake

The Best Software in the World on Aromatherapy!

Worldwide knowledge on 105 Essential Oils

- Pretty, Fun, and Easy to Use!
- Over 900 health conditions are covered in 3700 listings
- A slide show included to view many of the flowers
- Over 350 Actions and Properties of the oils
- Ten Thousand footnotes
- Free Editor so you can add your own wisdom
- Special notes, usage ideas, and warnings
- Information on 500 constituents of the essential oils
- Hundreds of alternate names from around the world

www.naturalhealthwizards.com
Designed for Windows from Win 95 to Win XP

Ayurvedic Remedies Software

by Steve Blake

Easy to Use and Quick to Learn!

Over 360 Ayurvedic Herbs and Remedies

Ayurvedic Remedies Software is a huge database of herbs and remedies from East Indian Ayurveda. Do your research on Ayurvedic remedies with this huge database of information from Indiaand around the world. Save time and find the secrets of the Ayurvedic tradition.

- Thousands of years of knowledge and tradition.
- Color photos bring the herbs to life
- Free Editor included for adding your own research.
- Herb summaries provide quick information.
- Thousands of unique conditions, actions and constituents.

www.naturalhealthwizards.com
Designed for Windows from Win 95 to Win XP

Chinese Patent Remedies Software

by Steve Blake

Your quick reference on Patent Remedies
68 Chinese Patent Remedies included

- ✦ Easy to Use, Quick to Learn.
- ✦ Covers the 68 Patent Remedies that are used the most.
- ✦ References to Jake Fratkin's book, *Chinese Herbal Patent Formulas*
- ✦ Almost 2000 listings of health conditions for easy look-up.
- ✦ Information is referenced to its source with over 4000 footnotes
- ✦ References to the *Clinical Handbook of Chinese Prepared Medicine* by Chun-Han Zhu
- ✦ Free Editor to add your own wisdom.
- ✦ References to the *Outline Guide to Chinese Herbal Patent Medicines* by Margaret Naeser
- ✦ Special notes, usage ideas, and warnings.
- ✦ Ingredients of the formulas usually include percentages — over 600 ingredients listings.
- ✦ Hundreds of alternate names to help you find the remedies.

www.naturalhealthwizards.com
Designed for Windows from Win 95 to Win XP